The
50 LIST

The
50 LIST
A father's heartfelt
message to his daughter

Anything is possible

NIGEL HOLLAND

HARPER

HARPER

An imprint of HarperCollins*Publishers*
77–85 Fulham Palace Road,
Hammersmith, London W6 8JB

www.harpercollins.co.uk

First published by HarperCollins*Publishers* 2013

1 3 5 7 9 10 8 6 4 2

© Nigel Holland 2013
Edited by Lynne Barrett-Lee
All photographs © Nigel Holland

Nigel Holland asserts the moral right to
be identified as the author of this work

A catalogue record of this book is
available from the British Library

ISBN 978-0-00-749324-1

Printed and bound in Great Britain by
Clays Ltd, St Ives plc

MIX
Paper from
responsible sources
FSC
www.fsc.org **FSC˙ C007454**

FSC™ is a non-profit international organisation established to promote
the responsible management of the world's forests. Products carrying the
FSC label are independently certified to assure consumers that they come
from forests that are managed to meet the social, economic and
ecological needs of present and future generations,
and other controlled sources.

Find out more about HarperCollins and the environment at
www.harpercollins.co.uk/green

For my darling wife, Lisa, and my wonderful children, Mattie, Amy and Ellie: with you beside me, I know anything is possible

Thanks also to my brothers, Mark and Gary, and my sister, Nicola: your love and support means everything to me

Finally, dear Mum and Dad: thanks for everything

'All men dream, but not equally. Those who dream by night in the dusty recesses of their minds, wake in the day to find that it was vanity: but the dreamers of the day are dangerous men, for they may act on their dreams with open eyes, to make them possible.'

T. E. LAWRENCE

INTRODUCTION

Just like any parent, I want the best for my children. I want them to feel safe, to be confident and to grow up with the understanding that life is to be challenged: to be explored and enjoyed, no matter what obstacles you might have to face. My wife and I have three great children and I am very proud of them. The two eldest, Matthew (15) and Amy (13), have grown up with responsibilities that most of their peers have never experienced. I am in a wheelchair, and being a wheelchair-using dad limits me from doing some of the things that other dads do, like football and cycling – activities that other parents take for granted. But their understanding of the issues I face makes the relationship I have with my children what it is: close, loving and, most of all, fun. They are growing up to be caring and thoughtful individuals with an empathy that belies their ages.

Ten years ago my wife, Lisa, gave birth to our youngest daughter, Eleanor. She has been diagnosed with the same condition that I have: Charcot-Marie-Tooth disease (CMT) or peroneal muscular atrophy, also known as hereditary motor and sensory neuropathy. What this means in practical terms is that there is wastage of the muscles in the lower part of the limbs. I can no longer walk and my hand strength is very weak, limiting my dexterity. Ellie is walking still but her gait – the way she walks – is affected. In 2010 she had to undergo surgery on her legs to try to straighten her ankles, as her tendons were pulling her feet inwards. The disability can affect people in many different ways.

Both my wife and I want to see Ellie enjoy life just as much as her older siblings and we are aware that she will face problems as she grows up, but what we want her to understand is that those problems can be overcome. In my life I have done many crazy and wonderful things that many people thought were beyond my capabilities: water-skiing, off-road 4x4, go-karting, gliding, diving – the list goes on. I even played drums in a band in the 1980s, reaching the dizzy heights of playing the Hippodrome at Leicester Square. Up until 2010 I was competing in the National Drag Racing Championships in a powerful Ford Mustang race car. I've never let anything stop me from realizing my dreams, so I want Ellie to know that her capabilities are to be explored. And it's not just that there's nothing wrong with 'having a go', either. It's that you'll never know what you can do till you try.

Then, one day, not so long ago, something else struck me: that there's a saying – or, more correctly, an idiom – that we all know, which goes 'actions speak louder than words'. And as soon as it occurred to me, that was it; I was away. I wouldn't just *tell* her. I would *show* her.

Nigel Holland, December 2012

SEPTEMBER

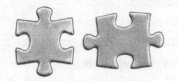

'Dad,' Ellie says to me, 'you're mad.'

'Well, you knew that already,' I say, grinning at the look of incomprehension on her face as she works her way down the piece of paper in her hand. It is a list. A list of all the crazy things I plan to do over the coming months. I can tell they're crazy just by looking at the expression on her face.

'Yeah, I know, Dad,' she says, 'but this is a big list. How are you going to do everything on it in one year?'

'I'm going to be doing even more than that,' I correct her. 'Because it's not finished yet. I was hoping you could suggest some things to put on it too.'

She looks again, her slender index finger tracing a line down the page. It's actually two lists, one marked 'extreme' and one marked 'other'. Ellie points to an item marked 'extreme'.

'What's this?' she asks.

'Zorbing?' I say, reading it. 'Oh, it's great fun. It's rolling down a hill inside a very large bouncy ball.'

She takes this in, and her look of incomprehension doesn't change. Though I've tried to explain to Ellie the main reason

why I'm doing this – to inspire her – Ellie has a learning difficulty, which means she doesn't always get the bigger picture.
But perhaps she doesn't need to. Not now, at least. All I really
want is that she gets caught up in the excitement and thinks
'can' rather than 'can't'. That'll be good enough for me. Though,
hmm, 'zorbing' – she's probably right: I *am* mad.

It's late in the afternoon, the watery late-September sun is
almost gone now, and we're contemplating what seemed like
a brilliant idea when I first thought of it, but which now seems
to mark me out as bonkers: a list of 50 challenges, of all kinds,
to be completed within the year, to prove that a) you really can
do almost anything that you put your mind to and b) turning
50 doesn't spell the end of any sort of life other than the pipe-
and-slippers kind.

Because that's what had struck me a couple of weeks earlier
when a work colleague had mentioned my upcoming 50th
birthday, saying that 50 – the *big* 50 – was a particularly
depressing milestone. One that marked the end of youth and
the beginning of 'being old', which was something I was not
prepared to be. 'And your point?' I'd retorted, rising swiftly to
the bait. 'I don't mind getting old, but I refuse to grow up.' It was
a thought – and a mindset – that had stayed with me all day.

And here we were, the idea having not only taken root but
also sprouted. And what had started as a whimsical, unfo-
cused kind of wish list had somehow become a full-blown
plan. A plan to prove something to both myself and my children – particularly my youngest, 'disabled' daughter.

'OK,' I say to Ellie. '*You* think of some challenges.'

She considers it for a few seconds, chewing thoughtfully

3

on her lower lip. 'Erm, maybe jump over a tall building?' she offers finally. And I'm pretty sure she's only half joking.

Which is nice – it's always good to be your children's superhero – but her idea is not do-able. Even for me. I say so.

'What about flying, then?' she says.

'What, you mean as in a plane?'

'No,' she retorts, in all seriousness. 'Like Superman!'

Silly me. I should have known. Of course she means like Superman. I am her hero, just the same way my dad was my hero. It's almost 30 years now since I lost him – over half a lifetime. And I still can't believe he's never coming back.

'Ah,' I tell Ellie, 'there's a problem with that one. I don't have any red underpants that will fit over my trousers.'

She knows she's being teased and pulls her 'Dad, I'm being teased' face. 'Well,' I say, 'you started it. What do you expect? But I can sort of fly,' I say, pointing to another item I've already added. 'Indoor skydiving. That's pretty much like flying.'

'What, you *can* fly?' She looks impressed now. 'What, with no strings or anything?'

'With no strings or anything. The air holds you up.' I try to explain how it works, but I'm not sure she quite gets it. 'Come on,' I say. 'What else? Think – what would you like to do, if you could do a challenge yourself?'

'Fly a kite,' she says, decisively. 'I'd like to fly a kite – a big pink one. Hey, but Dad?'

'What?'

'I've got a brilliant one for you. Dye your hair pink!'

She is bright eyed with excitement at this unexpected brainwave. Perhaps a little too bright eyed for my liking.

'Okaaayyy,' I say slowly. 'That can go under "maybe".'

Ellie shakes her head. 'You can't do maybes. You have to definitely promise.'

I try to regroup. How on earth am I going to get out of this one? The plan is to do all this stuff to inspire others, her included; not to look like a complete idiot, for a bet.

'I can't promise definitely,' I say. 'I might not have time to fit them all in, might I?'

'But if you do …'

'Then how about I put it on my "reserve list"?' I suggest. I have my clients to think about, after all. I write 'reserve list' on the bottom, followed by 'Dye hair pink'. Which her expression seems to suggest might have mollified her. 'Anything else?' I ask, trying to redirect her thoughts a bit. Which is probably tempting fate, but never mind.

'What about a puzzle?' she suggests.

'A jigsaw puzzle?'

'Yes. A jigsaw puzzle.'

'You know what, Ellie?' I say, already picking up my pencil. 'That is an excellent idea. Assuming you'll help me, of course.' I wiggle my fingers, which are probably cursing me already for the torture I am about to inflict on them.

'Course I'll help you,' she says. 'I'm brilliant at puzzles.'

'OK,' I say, adding it. 'How many pieces should we go for?'

'Five thousand,' she says, without a flicker of hesitation. 'That won't be too hard for your fingers, will it, Dad?'

'Piece of cake,' I tell my daughter. And at that point I believe it.

Mad. Just as Ellie has already said.

NOVEMBER

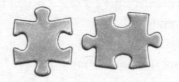

11 November 2011

Number of challenges still to be completed: 50.
Number of times I have wondered what I've let myself in for:
  Already too numerous to count.

Now I'm up and running with this thing, there's no backing out. No, I know I'm not exactly running yet – my plan is so far little more than a sketched-out idea – but having come up with it, I realize that committing to all these challenges is beginning to feel more and more like a challenge in itself. It's one thing telling yourself you're going to be able to achieve all of them, but quite another when you tell everyone else you are as well. Another still when the person you most want to do it for is one of the people dearest to you in the world.

As it turns out, I have been somewhat beaten off the blocks anyway, in terms of challenges, because only two weeks after formulating the plan, and my subsequent optimistic conversation with Ellie, I had another one lobbed into my lap. And it was a big one. A particularly big one for a man of my age.

After 13 happy years working as a web developer, I was made redundant from my job.

Sitting in the room that was once my study but has now been re-christened my 'office', in recognition of this new and exciting life stage, I think of Tommy Cooper and I smile. 'Just like that' – wasn't that his tag line? I was made redundant, just like that. At least that's the way it feels to me, though perhaps I should have seen it coming. Yet at the same time, I can't stop thinking about the timing of everything. Perhaps fate's played a part in all this happening when it has, because now nothing stands in the way of my doing what I've set out to do. I am all out of excuses. I have time on my hands. I also have a new item to add to my list of challenges: 'Make my business work.' Which is handy, because the zero gravity flight that it has now taken the place of was way too expensive to even begin to contemplate, and even more so for a guy with a family and a mortgage, but – crucially, and suddenly – without a job.

But it was definitely a job I'm going to miss. Though in recent years, after my firm was taken over by an American company, morale was low, stress was high and business was a bit shaky, the timing of the redundancy, in one sense, couldn't have been worse. During the last few months I was working for a really great manager, and though mostly from home – which was isolating, as I felt cut off from the office gossip – I felt energized about work in a way I hadn't in a long time, and I'm sad that it's all come to an end.

There was also the big question to face: how on earth would I pay the mortgage? But, though the simple option would be to take my skills and go and find another job with them, I had, and still have, a nagging sense that I should be taking the plunge and going it alone. Now or never. And I'm definitely less keen on never.

Which leaves me with now – do or die. Which is exciting yet scary.

So sending off my entry form for the Silverstone half marathon seems a little less daunting as a consequence. Though on the one hand it feels like one of the most difficult of all the challenges – 13 miles, and in a wheelchair: I am going to need to train and then some – when I compare it to the career cliff face I've just been forced to jump from (hoping to fly, obviously, rather than fall flat on my face) it feels suddenly more in the realms of the 'actually achievable': a solid thing, something I have control over.

As I sit at my desk filling in the online application form, I get a picture in my head of my beloved parents. Sadly, I don't have many pictures of them together. I have old, individual ones, taken with primitive cameras, black, white and sepia, and fluffy-edged with age. But nothing recent. Not many that show how much they loved one another. If I could change one thing in my life it would be that they could be here to see me do this. You never lose that feeling, I think, whatever your age.

*   *   *

According to family folklore, which is generally the most dubious kind, I always liked making an entrance. There must be some truth in it, though, because the story goes that when

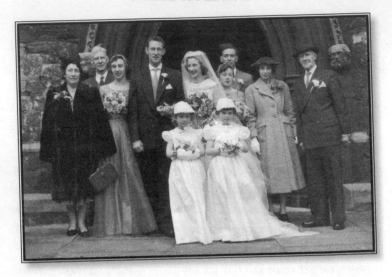

Mum and Dad's wedding.

I first looked like arriving, on 8 December 1962, my mother was busy serving dinner to no fewer than 12 guests.

To my perhaps unimaginative male eye, this seems quite a daring thing to be doing at any time, but particularly when you are 40 weeks pregnant. What became of the dinner guests and their dinners I don't know. All I do know is that I appeared several hours later, making landfall at Shrub Hill Hospital in Worcester, which was where my father had hastily relocated us. It's also said – more family folklore, this time probably 100 per cent reliable – that I was encouraged on my way by the irresistible smell of roast beef.

I was the third of three boys (which perhaps explains my mother's cool head in the face of a dozen hungry dinner guests), my brothers Mark and Gary then being six and four respectively. But I didn't keep my privileged position for very long. No sooner had I turned two than my world was disrupted – by the arrival of my baby sister, Nicola.

Nikki's arrival caused disruption in other ways as well. Unplanned, she came under the banner of 'unexpected gifts from heaven', but for me and my brothers she was anything but. We had wanted a dog. We had been promised a dog. Well, if not exactly promised, certainly given to believe that having a dog was not entirely out of the question. So for the duration of the pregnancy, we were miffed (though in my case, possibly still hopeful she might turn out to be a dog) and according to my mother, we spent the first six months of her life demanding that she be called Rover.

'Just as well you were a girl,' I recall my mother telling her later, 'or that might actually have turned out to be your name.'

The house the family lived in when I was born was in Britannia Square in Worcester. I have only a few memories of my time there. The house stood very tall, with three storeys, and was painted bright white. In my mind's eye, it was very grand looking, our family residence, though as a small child I naturally had a small child's perspective, so perhaps it wasn't quite as grand as it seemed.

Either way, it was home, and it was a happy home as well. Though my memories of it are no more than snapshots, I recall a wind-up mouse, which I wound and launched accidentally into my potty – the potty into which I'd just peed. I also have a clear early memory of my dad stepping out onto the roof of the house to sort out some tiling that had come loose. He was a jack of all trades, Dad – a builder, decorator

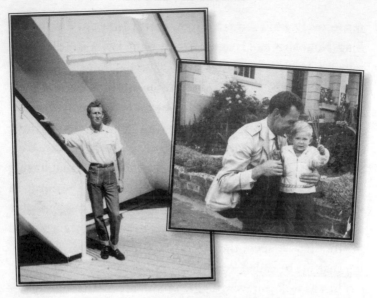

Left: My dad as a merchant seaman on board Merchant Ship Canberra.
Right: With my dad as a toddler.

and, at that time, a bus driver, and I can still recall how incredible it felt to look up and see him, high above my head, fixing the roof.

But then everything my dad did seemed incredible to me. I remember walking down the road with my mum, brothers and baby sister, and how we watched as a double-decker bus drove past us into the depot. Minutes later we had followed it – Mum had to deliver Dad's packed lunch to him – and I recall how thrilling it was to see my father climbing down from the cab of that very bus.

We didn't stay in Worcester for long. According to another piece of family folklore, my dad could drive anything – cars and buses, coaches and trucks, huge articulated lorries. If it had wheels and an engine, he was fine with it. As a result, within a couple of years of my sister's birth, Dad had found a new job. A better-paid one – which was key, given that he had a young and growing family – as a driver for BEA at Heathrow Airport.

We moved into a big sprawling semi in Hayes and Harlington, which was obviously convenient for Dad's work at the nearby airport, but was also elderly and in need of tart-

Left: The back of the house in Hayes and Harlington. The door led to the outside toilet – not good on a cold morning! Right: Gary, Mark and me digging in the front garden.

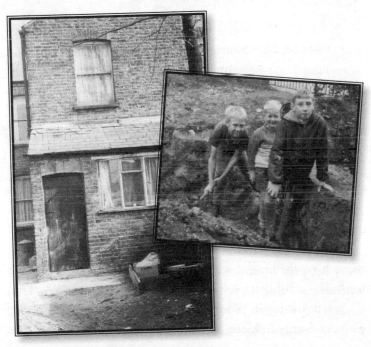

ing up. Which Dad of course did. Once again I have an enormous sense of pride in my father; he really did seem able to turn his hand to anything. Replacing windows, making furniture, painting walls, creosoting fences: there never seemed to be a day when he wasn't busy doing something. In the meantime, we kids played in the garden. This had an Anderson shelter, a relic of the Second World War, which, though it had long since been filled in with earth, provided us with our very own adventure playground: a grassy hummock to scramble over, a launch pad for our bikes, a backdrop for whatever games our young imaginations could conjure up.

*   *   *

Having sent in the entry form for the Silverstone half marathon, there is no turning back, and even if there were, I decide to seal the deal by announcing that I am taking part in it on Facebook, for good measure. As with telling all your mates you plan to give up smoking, putting it out there means there is NO WAY I can back out of it now.

For all my efficiency in telling the world what I'm up to, though, it's still going to be quite a leap of imagination to actually see myself completing a half marathon. And if my plan is to have any sort of credibility – not least with me – it's a leap I'd better start getting fit for.

Which means training. And training means several things must happen: hours of training itself, yes, but I must also cultivate a mindset of self-discipline and a big stock of dedication. Though in reality, I don't have a clue what I need to do to prepare. Note to self: so hurry up and find out!

DECEMBER

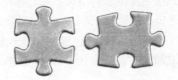

6 December 2011

Number of shopping days till Christmas: 19.
Number of days till my 49th birthday: 3.
Ergo, number of days till my 50th birthday: 368.
Number of challenges that need to be completed per day,
 therefore, on average: 0.137741.
Number of challenges that have actually been completed per
 day, on average: 0.000000.

Well, I've been busy training, haven't I? I have just, in fact, returned from a 5-mile training lap around the town. And I have decided upon a new motivational slogan: if I can make it around Wellingborough, I can make it anywhere. (Which will obviously, of necessity, include Silverstone.) No, it doesn't have quite the same ring as the lyric from 'New York, New York', but it is what I believe to be true.

It's all about motivation, obviously. The way the weather is looking right now, I might not get another chance to get out and train till after Christmas, so it feels good to have got the laps I have done in the bag. Admittedly, a half marathon is 13 miles, not 5, but in terms of conditions there's no contest. What with the state of the roads and pavements, pot holes, broken kerbs – not to mention countless badly parked cars – just negotiating the route of my training lap is a major challenge. It's also pretty hilly, which, in a wheelchair, is hard on the arms, so all things considered (and wheeling round, I've had plenty of time to consider) 13 miles on a perfectly smooth, level racetrack doesn't daunt me quite so much now.

I Skype my brother Gary, who lives just outside Frankfurt in Germany. He studied performance sports at school and still plays squash at a high level, so is the ideal person to give me training tips and encouragement. He tells me to eat carbs, drink plenty of water, practise having a positive mental attitude and generally live a life of such wholesome sobriety till March that as soon as we're done I feel a compulsion to crack open a large beer.

10 December 2011

Number of years on the planet now: 49. And I don't feel a day older than 77 (post-training complications – i.e. I hurt).
Number of challenges completed: Erm … still have not quite done any yet.
However, bottles of good Merlot consumed: 1.

I was 49 yesterday, and the thing that most sticks in my mind is that I now have just 364 days to complete all 50 challenges, or else I am going to look something of an idiot. It was a nice birthday – though we dubbed it something different. As Lisa and I dined from the Christmas lunchtime menu at the Beckworth Garden Emporium (and why not? They have a cracking restaurant) we decided we'd call it the Mantisweb staff Christmas party, Mantisweb being the name I've given my new business. Which of course gave us licence to misbehave generally, though neither of us actually photocopied our bottoms.

My birthday over – Christmas isn't allowed to begin until it is – the festivities are coming around super-fast now, and Lisa and I still don't know what to get the kids. With all my redundancy pay already allocated to pay the mortgage, money's tight, so it's not going to be an extravagant affair this year. I find I don't see that as a bad thing, particularly. Perhaps it's good to keep things a little simpler – more like the Christmases of my own youth, when there were only three TV channels, there was no 24/7 scheduling, and a snowball wasn't just something you lobbed at your mates but some foul, yellow, frothy thing your mum drank. Well, my mum did, anyway, and whichever way you look at it, I can't help but look back at Christmases past and wish Christmases present were just a little more like them.

*   *   *

Despite us having very little materially then, compared to today's festive excesses, it really did feel like a time of plenty. It was a time when not only did the dustmen get a crate of brown ale from Dad, as an annual thank you, but also the

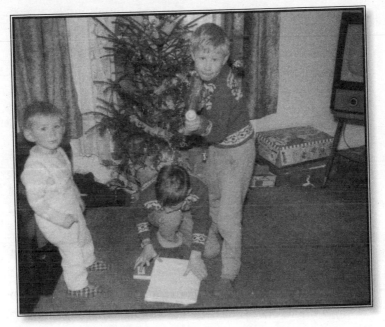

Christmas time at the Holland house.

entire contents of the drinks cabinet (actually the sideboard) were brought out on top, dusted off and arranged, like a help-yourself bar at a wedding reception. It was a time of corner-to-corner paper streamers in the living room and glittering skeins of tinsel for the tree. Which was, of course, a real one.

It's a cliché now, but we did all really get tangerines in our stockings, plus chocolate (festive chocolate, obviously: golden coins, or Lindt kittens) and a pack of playing cards or some little toy. I remember one year getting a yoyo and not having a clue what to do with it, so I just swung it round and round my head, nearly taking out the light fittings.

The presents done – a military exercise, involving four piles, four anxious children and then one unholy scramble – we children would accompany Dad, playing family postman, delivering gifts to all our relatives while Mum got on with lunch. And what a lunch it was, because Mum was a fantastic cook, and made the best onion bread sauce on the planet, bar none.

The drink of choice on Christmas Day *chez* the Hollands was Pomagne. A poor man's champagne, made from cider, it felt like the height of sophistication – or would have, had Dad been more adept at handling it. It was always a tense moment when he attempted to get the cork out, ever since the year when it flew out, headed for the ceiling at great velocity, came back down and landed in the gravy boat, propelling most of its contents all over my brother Mark.

Lunch over – and perhaps as a result of the Pomagne – Mum would always tell her annual Christmas joke. Which was a pretty ropey one, but, in keeping with the spirit of the occasion, we didn't care: we'd roll about at every telling.

Mum: 'What did the elephant say when the mouse ran up its trunk?'

Us: 'We don't know. What *did* the elephant say when the mouse ran up its trunk?'

Mum (pinching her nose hard together with her thumb and forefinger and speaking in a squeaky voice): 'Hmm! I suppose you think that's funny!'

You're right. You probably had to be there.

But for all the joy of my childhood, it wasn't without its worries. Though I was unaware of it, my parents were becoming anxious about me. I must have been around three or four when they first started noticing problems with my toes. They would curl up every time I tried to put my feet into my wellington boots. I was OK with shoes and sandals, but there was something about the angle your foot is at when you feed it into a wellington boot that gave me problems. Once my toes were inside, I couldn't seem to straighten them out by myself. My parents also noticed that my gait wasn't quite natural; I would walk in a way that perhaps I would today describe as 'hopeful', flicking my lower legs forward, rather than placing them as you would normally, in the hope that the heel would hit the ground before the toes did. If the latter happened (and as I grew, this became more and more evident), the result – flat on my face – sure wasn't pretty.

I had no idea how much this concerned them, obviously. My toes did what they did, and my gait was what it was. I felt no frustration about any of this; I just worked around it. I was only little, after all. I knew no different.

I had other things on my mind, in any case. While Mum and Dad tried to rationalize their concerns by saying my problems were just part of me 'growing up', I was much more concerned with that other big growing-up thing: not being a baby any more, I couldn't wait to start school. With two big brothers already there, I was aching to join the party. I didn't want to be stuck at home with only my little sister for company; I wanted to be where the big boys were.

When my brother Gary announced one morning that today was the day, my excitement at going knew no bounds. But I was destined for disappointment. The first disappointment was the news, once we arrived there, that I wouldn't be joining my big brothers in the junior school as I'd expected. I would have to go elsewhere – well, a whole playground away, anyway – as I was only old enough, apparently, to join the infants. The second disappointment was that as soon as Mum left, all my confidence went scuttling away with her. Within the space of a few hours I'd had all the stuffing knocked out of me; I felt anxious, alone and very lost.

Thankfully, the feeling didn't last. In fact, another revelation was that the business of making friends there was unexpectedly straightforward, and seemed to consist of the simplest of exchanges.

'This your first day?' a boy said.

'Yes,' came my mumble.

'OK. Wanna play football?'

Job done.

Best of all was that it seemed to work with almost everyone (bar the girls, of course). You played football with someone and you had a friend for the rest of your natural life. Or at least for the immediate future, till the bell went, which, as with any four-year-old, was as far ahead as I generally thought.

But the problems with my curling toes weren't going away and had now started to impact on my getting dressed for school. It had begun to take me so long that Mum even began stressing that I'd become phobic about going for some reason.

Nothing could have been further from the truth. I loved school. But certain aspects of it were becoming more challenging for me, clearly. And though, once again, I wasn't really aware of this myself, my parents became increasingly concerned. Their concern mostly centred on my gait. I didn't walk like my siblings and no one knew why – and my gait definitely wasn't getting better. After a couple of months of this, my mother made her mind up: she would take me to the local clinic to see a doctor.

I still remember my incomprehension about this visit. I wasn't feeling sick, and nor did I have a sore throat or a rash, but even so, I was being taken out of lessons. Why was that? I was no less confused when we got there and the doctor immediately took off my shoes and socks and began tapping my ankles with a little rubber hammer.

But it was my mum who was most confused when, the foot inspection over, the doctor turned his attention to my arms and hands. She was just about to ask him what my hands had to do with anything when he let out a loud and alarming 'Hmmmm …'

'What?' asked Mum anxiously.

'Hmmm …' said the doc again. 'I think young Nigel here needs to go and see a specialist.'

He then began talking over my head, to my mum, while she helped me put my shoes and socks back on. I didn't understand much of what he was saying – though I soon would – but the gist of it seemed clear: 'I don't actually have a clue what's wrong with your son, Mrs Holland, so I'll pack him off to someone who might.'

On the way home, feeling as you do after a visit to the doctor (a little bit relieved, a lot brave, a tad martyred), I hoped – even expected – that there might be something in it for me. A small toy perhaps, a bag of sweets, a penny lollipop. But I got nothing. Mum was never one for over-indulging her kids. I got deposited straight back at school.

FEBRUARY

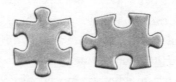

8 February 2012

Number of inches of snow dumped on Wellingborough in
*   January: Easy – more than enough to prevent me from*
*   getting out.*
Ergo, number of challenges so far completed: Still 0.
However, number of challenges attempted today (finally):
*   1 – 'Donate blood.'*
But number of challenges actually completed today: Another
*   big fat 0. Oh, and I also got wet.*

Well, that was a great start, I don't think. You might have
noticed that, despite a flurry of early enthusiasm and activity,
there is nothing recorded here for January. Which is because
nothing actually happened in January. Yup, that's correct.
Nothing whatsoever. Yes, we ate, slept and did all the day-to-
day things that needed doing, but in terms of My Big
Important Project, not a thing.

I know I shouldn't beat myself up too much. The bottom
line is that wheelchairs and snow do not mix – unless you

count regularly landing on your own bottom line among your list of favourite pastimes. And it's not as if I haven't been getting things under way, making phone calls, sending emails and doing research.

But I'm frustrated because apart from signing up for the half marathon (which does not mean actually doing it, of course, however many training laps I put in before Christmas), becoming a blood donor was to have been pretty much my first completed challenge, and the one I was most keen to get over with.

Except I haven't got it over with. Which is infuriating, as the day began so positively. Well, I say positively, but there wasn't really anything positive about it. Just naked fear. Because actually I was terrified.

'So why are you doing it, then, Dad?' Ellie wanted to know. It was a reasonable enough question. Though I was pretty sure that by now she understood the concept of the list and why I was doing it, I wasn't so sure she'd embraced the idea that it might include doing things I didn't want to do.

We were all finishing breakfast, before the kids left for school. Though I say 'we', I couldn't eat a thing, because I was off to become a blood donor in less than an hour, the thought of which had completely robbed me of my appetite.

'Because I'm confronting my fears,' I said, probably rather grandly, in an attempt, as much as anything, to psyche myself up for it. 'That's what you do,' I went on. 'That's what makes it a challenge. That it's difficult is really the whole point. If it was easy for me, it wouldn't be challenging, would it? If it was

Mum doing it, say,' (Lisa's a long-term blood donor) 'it would be easy. But because I have a phobia –'

Ellie looked confused now. 'What's a phobia?'

'An irrational fear,' Matt supplied. 'Like when you're really scared of snakes or spiders –'

'There is nothing irrational about being scared of snakes and spiders,' Amy chipped in. 'Not if they're cobras or rattle-snakes or black widows or something …'

'And yours is needles?' Ellie asked. 'Needles being poked in your arm?' She demonstrated on herself for me. 'And then sucking all your blood out …' she added, warming to the idea now. 'A bit like they're *vampires*?'

Which wasn't the best image to be starting the day with, frankly. *Twilight* has an awful lot to answer for.

'Not like vampires,' said Lisa, presumably seeing I was turning green now. 'Nothing at all like vampires, in fact. No, it's done by nurses, and they're very, very gentle. Dad will hardly feel a thing, because they're also *very* good at it …'

But still a lot like vampires, even so.

*   *   *

It's not surprising that I have a phobia of needles. From the age of five, and throughout my childhood, they were coming at me from all angles.

My first foray into a world that would become painfully familiar happened just a few weeks after my visit to the GP, when a letter arrived requesting my presence at an appointment that had been made for me at Guy's Hospital in London.

Being so small still, I didn't have much idea what was happening. Though I'm sure Mum and Dad told me, I have no memory of making a connection between my bendy toes and the trip to the big city. Going to London was, and would continue to be, synonymous with only one thing for me: a trip to go and visit my Auntie Betty.

My aunt and uncle lived in a sprawling housing estate just off Abbey Road, and I'd go and stay with them at least once every summer. I loved going to visit Auntie Betty and Uncle Gerry. Together they ran a successful stock car racing team, which made them terribly exciting to be with. They would travel all around the country, to race their car in the national championships, and we'd set off to whichever venue we were headed for in an enormous coach that they'd converted from the standard passenger variety into something that, in its day, would not have seemed out of place in a Formula 1 paddock. It carried the stock car on the back and the inside had been adapted so that we could not only sit in it but also sleep in it.

Trips to Auntie Betty's were the genesis of what would become a lifelong passion for motorsport, and from a very early age, one of the highlights of travelling to London was the point when we'd go through a long tunnel on the A4, and I got that tingle of anticipation, knowing we'd soon be there.

This was different, though. And the big difference that sticks in my mind was that rather than end up at Auntie Betty's, as usual, we arrived at a scary place, full of incredibly high buildings. In reality not so enormous – hardly the Manhattan skyline – but to little me, they seemed so tall that they blocked out the sun. There was noise, too – so much noise. So many car engines, and bus engines – so many horns blaring all at once, as if all the traffic on the roads was really angry.

And barking. I clearly recall the noise of dogs barking. Strange, looking back – we were nowhere near Battersea – but that's always stuck in my mind.

I also have a vivid mental picture of the inside of the hospital. And an equally clear one of the great men I was about to meet. I had been summoned to see two eminent physicians of the day: a brace of consultants called the McArdle brothers, who were leaders in the field of neuroscience.

My main impression, not surprisingly for those days, was of brown. Unlike the clinically white environments you find in most modern hospitals, the office of the McArdle brothers was a symphony of dark wood: heavy wooden filing cabinets – the contents of each drawer identified with its own white, handwritten label; dark-wood chairs – one for each of them, plus a further three ordinary, dark, school chairs for me, Mum and Dad; and a hefty dark-wood desk with an inlaid leather top. Looking back, the only thing missing from the tableau was a couple of those globe-shaped glass bottles full of brightly coloured water whose function was, and still is, a mystery.

Also in keeping with the fashion of the time, the McArdle brothers – looking rather frightening in their matching white coats – puffed merrily on cigarettes before mounting their attack. I had come to be investigated and they went at it with gusto, putting me through a series of increasingly scary tests. I was prodded and poked, inspected and injected, and at the end of it, the brothers reached their professional conclusion.

Mum and Dad had been right: there was definitely something wrong with me. I had some sort of hereditary muscle-wasting condition, apparently, and to be sure they would need to do some tests.

Everything changed for my parents that day. And, looking back, I'm not surprised; it must have come as such a shock. Though the condition was apparently hereditary, there was no history of it in either family, meaning that it must be the result of some random mutant gene.

We returned home, and while I carried on doing all the things little boys did, largely oblivious to my 'condition', they could only look on as my muscles became progressively weaker and – having no experience or medical knowledge of what was wrong with me – worry about what the future might hold for me.

Not that my childhood, from that day, was really normal. Though Mum and Dad never allowed me to dwell on whatever it was that was causing my problems (if I became tired after playing, then I rested, but they never stopped me doing anything), it increasingly impacted on my life. This was mostly because life began to be punctuated by interruptions: an endless round of hospital visits, while they tried to better understand what was causing my symptoms. There was obviously no choice but to put up with it all, but hospitals – and everything that seemed to happen within them – soon became the bane of my life. I disliked all of it – in fact, 'dread' probably isn't too strong a word here. What child wants to be in and out of hospital, dragged away from his friends and whatever fun things they might be up to? I particularly hated the seemingly endless in-patient visits to the Hillingdon Hospital and the National Hospital for Neurology and Neurosurgery in Queen Square. Both places soon filled me with anxiety and fear. And much of the reason for that was that I soon learned I couldn't trust them. They would say one thing – normally a nice, reassuring thing – and then the exact opposite would happen.

A particularly grim time was at the hospital in Queen Square, where, aged seven, I had to have some nerve induction tests. These tests, which I had to have a number of times, involved an electrode being attached to my ankle, and a needle, with a wire attached, put into my thigh. They would then pass a small electric current through the electrode, so that they could assess the strength of the signal in my peripheral nerves by picking up the signal in the wire.

I think I sort of understood why they needed to do it, but what I never got my head around was what they said every time.

'Now, Nigel, this won't hurt,' they'd confidently assure me 'All that will happen is that your leg muscle will sort of "jump".'

Which it duly did. But what I never seemed to be able to get across to them (and how nice it is to be able to make this point here) was that it was my leg, and actually it did hurt!

As I was so young, and an 'inmate', which was sort of how it worked back then, the doctors would gather around my bed and talk over me and about me, and, without my parents around to explain what was happening, my only source of information about what horrors might be inflicted next came by way of updates from the nurses after the ward rounds.

'They're going to take you to occupational therapy,' I remember one telling me during one stay, 'to be assessed,' she finished mysteriously. It meant absolutely nothing. What on earth was 'occupational therapy?' I could hardly pronounce it, and like all the other unpronounceable words they bandied about, I didn't like the sound of it one bit.

'What are they going to do to me?' I wanted to know. 'Does it involve "tests"?'

'Tests' was a word I *could* pronounce, but I was anxious about them too. Because experience had taught me that tests almost always seemed to involve needles in some way. 'No, not at all,' she replied. 'Really. It's nothing to worry about, Nigel.'

But her reassurance, helpful though it was, was short-lived. 'And after that,' she added quickly (presumably thinking that if she slipped it in I might not notice), 'they're going to take you off to have a lumbar punch.'

This was a new one. And one that I definitely didn't like the sound of. As soon as the nurse elaborated, I was terrified. OK, so it turned out that it didn't involve being punched by a tree trunk, but what it did involve – in essence, being punctured by an extremely large needle – sounded even more terrifying. A lumbar puncture is when a needle is inserted into your spinal cord and a small amount of spinal fluid drawn off. And as I lay on the bed, curled into a tight ball – knees to chest, as instructed – I was as petrified of that needle as I could be.

'All over soon,' the nurse kept saying, patting my head.

'And you won't feel a thing,' the doctor helpfully reassured me, 'because I'm going to anaesthetize the area first.' And, to give him his due, on this occasion he was right. Apart from the initial prick – which obviously I did feel – I felt absolutely nothing, and the only bad bit was afterwards when I had to lie on my back for 24 hours, while enduring the worst headache of my young life.

Much worse, in terms of my increasing phobia, was the endless round of blood tests I seemed to have at Hillingdon Hospital, which was staffed by a rogue gang of vampire medics – it must have been, because harvesting my blood seemed to be a favourite pastime. Looking back, I suppose their fascination with looking at it was for a valid reason: I had an extremely rare disease, which they were researching all the time, and I made an excellent guinea pig and pin cushion.

When I was growing up, little was known about CMT. It affects some 23,000 people in the UK and research into it was a vital step in the process of learning how to manage its manifestations. These are many: foot drop, chronic tiredness, bone abnormalities, muscle atrophy, balance issues, loss of dexterity, fatigue and chronic pain. Though I didn't know all this as a little boy, obviously, I still felt I had to agree to being a guinea pig. Saying no wasn't an option – not if I wanted to better deal with my disease. The doctors and scientists needed to know about it and, more importantly, so did Mum and Dad.

My poor parents. While as a child I had to deal with its many inconveniences, they had the unenviable task of steering me through a childhood and adolescence knowing that my nerve function would gradually deteriorate and that I'd more than likely end up with a major disability. They had to cope with the knowledge of what might be ahead for me.

But it was hard to be that guinea pig, however much I knew I had to. The medics took blood from me at any opportunity they got, and with every needle they stuck into my arms, my fear grew – so much so that one day it took three nurses and a doctor to hold me down, so that they could get their standard inch of glistening fluid. 'Well done!' they'd say. 'There we are! That didn't hurt at all, did it?'

Erm, yes. Yes it did hurt. A lot.

And it didn't just hurt: it became a source of constant anxiety. Like any other child, I loved my parents and wanted to please them. They were trying to make sense of something no one understood, and naturally – and quite rightly – put their trust in the doctors and scientists who were just starting to get to grips with what CMT was. And having me as a real-life case study (either willing or unwilling) was a central part of amassing the vital information that would, everyone hoped, make my life less challenging. So I would never dream of criticizing my parents for the years of investigations I had to go through. They were doing their best for me. They never did anything less than their best for me. Just as Lisa and I want to do our very best for Ellie. Though thank goodness she's been born into another time.

*   *   *

The kids duly dispatched to their various places of learning, Lisa and I cleared the kitchen and then headed into Wellingborough, to the church hall where I had my date with destiny.

Apart from the constant nausea, the sweating palms and the gnawing terror, I was actually feeling quite well prepared.

I had done my research. I'd often read about the whole 'confront your fears' approach to dealing with a phobia, and had been impressed by the case studies of chronic arachno-phobics who, after doing just that, had been completely trans-formed and would let tarantulas skip merrily along their arms. Encouraged, I'd been for a browse on the NHS website, and, having chatted on the phone to a very helpful lady about the process, and having also covered the potential complications of my disability, I had already registered as a first-time donor.

Today, then, was the culmination of a serious purpose. After all, this wasn't just about ticking an item off a list. It was about doing it for that warm glow of pride in an achievement – to enjoy the thought that my blood would be going to help someone somewhere; I'd confront my fear *and* I'd do good. What better example could there be for Ellie?

Even so, as we pulled up outside the church where the mobile service was, all I could think of was how fervently I wanted to just get in, give the blood and then get the hell out of there.

'You'll be fine,' Lisa said reassuringly, as I parked the car in the church car park. She'd been saying it at regular intervals since we'd got up that morning, and though I was grateful – Lisa's always such a big support when I'm feeling anxious – her reassurance was falling on deaf ears. I probably *would* be fine, I knew that, but that's the thing with phobias: you think one thing, but your body does another.

The weather wasn't helping much, either. There was heavy snow forecast over the coming days, and, perhaps as a taster, or perhaps as a personal portent, heavy rain had fallen overnight. And because a car had parked close to the ramped kerb I needed, my only way into the church was via a deep muddy puddle. Not something that would normally faze me – I'm quite an expert in my wheelchair – but, given the circumstances and my growing sense of impending doom, wheeling wetly through it (while busy cursing inconsiderate parkers everywhere) only added to my sense of foreboding.

Inside the church hall, where the temporary blood-letting – sorry, blood donor – service had been set up, there was little to cling onto that would reassure the average phobic. Seven gurneys, I counted, once I'd given my name and we'd transferred to the waiting area, and on each was a compliant donor, to whom was attached a needle, which was attached to a tube, which fed the donor's blood, in regular deep-red drips, into a plastic bottle. If there was ever a point to turn tail, this was definitely it; but strangely, though it looked like a scene from *Doctor Who*, there was something about the vampires – sorry, nurses – who were running this particular show that made the whole scene look unexpectedly calm and peaceful. And as a bonus, there was no one actually screaming. To my surprise, I felt a sense of relative calm begin to descend.

'You'll be fine,' Lisa whispered again, seeing my gaze and misreading the effect it was all having on me.

'You know what?' I whispered back (it was that kind of place – hush felt obligatory). 'I am actually looking forward to doing this, now we're in here.'

'You are?' She didn't look convinced.

But there was no time to wax lyrical about my new-found inner calm, because my name was called then, and we went off to a small temporary cubicle, where a nurse bearing a biro wanted to know all about my condition. This was a surprise, as it had been discussed at some length on the phone, as well as being detailed on the registration form.

Risking a quip, I explained that my 'condition' was 'sitting down', which she obviously found so unfunny that she went to great lengths to explain that since she personally didn't know anything about my real condition, she couldn't take blood from me without a letter from my doctor.

'But I'm absolutely fine to do that,' I explained. 'I'm not ill.' I explained again that this had already been covered over the phone.

But she was having none of it. As they didn't know that, even if I did, I would need to get the letter before they could risk taking blood from me. And that was the end of it. I would have to go away and then come back again the next time the blood donor service was in town.

'Isn't there any way around this?' I asked her. 'Coming here's been a really big thing for me today. It's one of my challenges, you see.' I told her about my 50 List, half hoping she might have seen it in the local paper; I explained how it worked, and what I was doing it for. 'And this one's particularly dear to me,' I finished, 'because of my phobia of needles. I've had it since I was a child, and I was determined to beat it. Meet it head on –'

But I could tell from her expression that there was no way I'd be meeting it today. 'You have a phobia?' she said. 'Oh, well, in that case, we wouldn't take your blood anyway.'

Apparently they felt it wasn't a very good way of ridding someone of a phobia. So that was that. They all apologized, and I wheeled myself out again, my needle phobia still there to fight another day.

'Never mind,' said Lisa as we drove home, mission not accomplished. 'You'll just have to think of a new challenge to replace it. There'll be something ...'

We lapsed into what we hoped would be a productive, thoughtful silence.

And it was. An idea suddenly came to me. 'I'll try wood turning.'

'Wood turning?' Lisa asked. 'Where on earth did that come from?'

'Erm ... it's dexterous? It involves using my fingers? It's probably tricky?'

Definitely tricky, if my childhood exploits in woodwork class are anything to go by.

'And there's a thought,' I said testily. 'Let's hope I don't rip my finger off on the lathe and require pints and pints of blood to save me, eh?'

Lisa smiled. 'You'll be fine,' she said firmly.

14 February 2012

Number of challenges still to be completed: Er ... still 50.
But number of challenges that are almost definitely going to be happening less than 10 days from now, all at once, and ON THE BBC no less: A big fat 3! Hurrah! Now we're talking.

Just put down the phone to a man called Matt Ralph. He is a BBC television producer. Am *amazed*. What a difference a day can make, eh?

Everyone makes New Year resolutions, don't they? Give up drink. Lose a stone. Read *War and Peace*. Be a Better Person. But having already made 50 of them before Christmas – way more than most people – come the New Year, I didn't need to do much resolving. No, what I needed to do was get on and actually *do* them, and suddenly here we were, edging into spring, and barely anything had yet been done, bar a failed attempt to get someone to take some blood. I was beginning to feel that my deadline, 9 December 2012, my 50th birthday, was breathing down my neck.

I hadn't even been able to get out and do much training for the half marathon, my initial burst of enthusiasm having been rained on from a great height. Frozen rain, in fact: the much forecasted, much anticipated and now interminable snow. And there are only so many times you can make a circuit of the coffee table before losing the will to live and/or becoming so dizzy you pass out.

'You need publicity,' my friend Simon Cox said to me firmly. It was a Tuesday, the kids were in school, and he was over to discuss business. He was a client now, as well as a close pal of mine, and once we were done discussing e-commerce solutions for his company, I'd showed him the new 50 List website I'd created – my pet project once the kids had gone back to school.

I'd also by now set up a JustGiving account. My mentioning the list on Facebook had brought a flurry of enquiries from friends wanting to know where and how they could make donations – and, more importantly, who I wanted to have them. So it made sense to make things official by putting that information on the website too, explaining that anyone who felt inspired to could donate direct to CMT United Kingdom, the charity that was the first port of call for people with CMT, myself obviously very much included. The money would then be split equally between ongoing research and supporting youngsters, like Ellie, with the condition.

I'd set myself a pretty ambitious target as well – to raise £5,000.

'I know,' I said to Simon. 'It's a lot to aim for, isn't it?'

'Which is why you need to get it out there,' he said. 'Fire people's imaginations about it. Give them a chance to get involved. Local businesses even, maybe. It's the sort of thing the local papers will jump on too, believe me. That might lead to sponsorship – financial help and so on.' He pointed to some of the more outlandish challenges I'd set myself. 'Which, by the look of this, you're really going to need.'

Perhaps because I'd always thought I'd fund the list myself, it had never occurred to me to involve the local papers in what I was doing. I said so.

'Are you mad?' Simon laughed. 'It's January, remember – nothing doing. They'll be all over this, trust me. Take a look out of the window. I reckon they'll leap on any story they can lay their hands on right now that doesn't need to include the word "snow".'

I did as instructed and agreed he was probably right. *I'd* leap on anything that didn't involve snow at the moment.

Much as I didn't want to be a grump and a killjoy, snow and wheelchairs were incompatible: that was a fact of life.

'Seriously,' he went on, 'they'll be all over this *anytime*. Tell you what. I have a friend who knows a journalist down at the *Herald and Post*. Let me have a word with her. See if she can get him to do a piece on it. Spread the word a bit for you. How about that?'

'You think?' I said. 'You really think he'll be that interested in all this?'

Simon grinned. 'Nige, mate, you really don't know what you've got here, do you? Just you wait and see, mate. Just you wait.'

And it wasn't a very long wait. It was around 24 hours, give or take – no more than that – before a journalist from the *Herald and Post* was indeed on the phone wanting to talk to me and, having asked me a few questions about what I was up to, wanting to know when he could send their photographer round and get some pictures of both me and, he hoped, Ellie.

She was typically bemused at the prospect of being in the paper.

'But why?' she kept asking on the morning of the shoot. 'Shoot' – in itself a heck of a concept to get my head around.

'So that everyone can hear about what I'm doing and why I'm doing it,' I explained to her. 'To spread the word, and I hope raise money for CMT.'

'Yes,' she said, 'but why do they want a picture of *me*?'

'Because you're one of the main reasons Dad wants to do it,' explained Lisa. She was brandishing a duster with an expression of mild fanaticism. She had been all morning.

Where dust was concerned, she'd be taking no prisoners. There was no way her living room would be featured in the local paper looking anything less than squeaky clean and perfect. I wouldn't have been surprised to be given a quick buff and polish myself. She'd already given the dog the once-over.

'But you don't have to if you don't want to,' I added quickly. Although I was doing this to inspire my youngest daughter, there was no way I was going to make her do something she didn't want to do. So if she didn't want to do it, then so be it. Ellie is feisty and self-possessed, but she is also quite shy. And the last thing I wanted was for any of this to make her stressed, or for her to feel that she was being pushed into the limelight.

But she surprised me. 'OK,' she said. 'I don't mind. It might be cool.' Then she hurried off upstairs to get changed into her favourite Minnie Mouse T-shirt.

Then, as they probably became sick and tired of saying in the papers that particular winter, the whole thing, to our amazement, snowballed. The piece appeared in the paper the next day – it even had its own front-page intro – and the phone, as a consequence, began ringing.

First it was a news agency, SWNS, who expressed great enthusiasm for handling my 'story', which was something I'd never even thought of it as. It was a project, my project, that was all. But they disagreed. It was very much a story, they told me, and one they were keen to put out to the nationals, to see what they might make of it, too.

So they did, and they came back to me the following morning to tell me that it had also now been published in *Metro*, the *Sun*, the *Daily Mirror* and the *Daily Telegraph*. Not huge pieces

– only a few column inches in most cases – but I was flabbergasted, as was Lisa, and all the kids.

The days that followed were no less surreal. In fact, they rank among the craziest and most overwhelming I've ever experienced.

Next came the calls from various radio stations. Would I be prepared to talk about The 50 List on air? Absolutely.

Then magazines. Would I be prepared to do interviews with them? Naturally. Then TV – 5 News, to be precise. Would I be prepared to travel down to London to be on their programme and tell the world how the idea of The 50 List had come about?

By now the phone was ringing almost constantly. No sooner had I hung up on yet another enthused researcher, and gone into the kitchen to give Lisa the latest update, than – brinngg brinnggg! – straight away it rang again.

'Can you believe this?' I asked Lisa every time it started up again. 'So this is what 15 minutes of fame feels like, is it?' I'd never dealt with anything quite so manic in my life

Happily, the news agency stepped in to help us out, and became the contact to whom I could direct all the callers. This left me and Lisa free to think about what we could and couldn't do.

The reality was that going down to London, to Channel 5, would be something of a mission. It would mean an incredibly early start and a complex journey via public transport; and both the prospect and the expense were a bit daunting. But it would potentially be a brilliant way to help my cause – and, I hoped, help me reach my fundraising target. Should I go?

I was still dithering when the email came in this morning – the email that topped them all. The big one.

Hi Nigel,

I'm a director working for *The One Show* at the BBC. I read an article about you and your daughter Eleanor in today's *Metro*. I was sorry to read about your daughter's diagnosis but it sounds like you are doing something really amazing to inspire her.

I wondered if I might be able to find out more about your challenges with the view of possibly helping you set up and complete some of them and film a piece about it for *The One Show*? If this sounds like something you might be interested in please feel free to get in touch. I'll be happy to answer any questions and we can discuss what is possible and what is not.

Thanks for your time and hope to hear from you soon.

Best,

Karolina

I got straight on the phone, which was how I got to talk to Matt Ralph. And though I still can't quite believe it, it's all fixed. On 23 February I get to complete not one but *three* of my challenges: I'm going to do an indoor skydive, take a 4x4 off road and go powerboating as well. Now we're not only talking the talk, as they say, we're walking the walk, too. Well, sort of.

*   *   *

Not every test I had during my childhood involved needles and pain. Sometimes the tests were just very odd. One time, when I was around 14, I was summoned back to the National Hospital for Neurology and Neurosurgery in Queen Square, London, where they wanted to glue a load of electrodes to my head, which would then be connected to a large machine. Naturally, by now, I was wary of anything that anyone in a white coat did, so it took the doctor some time to convince me not only that he wasn't going to kill me but also that there wouldn't be any pain involved.

'You won't feel a thing,' he kept telling me. 'You can't. Because brains can't feel pain – did you know that? All that's going to happen is that the machine is going to read all the messages that your optic nerve sends to it.'

Which sounded worrying in itself, but I had no choice other than to go along with it, and sat patiently while he prepared me for his investigations. First he used a chinagraph pencil and a tape measure to make marks on my scalp where the electrodes needed to go. He followed this up with globs of glue, to which he stuck small white discs, to which he then connected a load of wires. These wires, around a dozen of them (one for every disc), were connected to a large (and I do mean large) metal cabinet, the front of which was a sea of lights, dials, switches and oscilloscopes, none of which, he hastened to add – once I was finally connected to it, and frankly terrified – were out to do me any harm.

The only harm done that day was to my sanity. I had to stare at a moving dot in the middle of a chequered board, and that was it. Nothing else. For an hour. I've never sat and watched paint dry, but I imagine the two are similar. Certainly my dad, who was supposed to be there for moral support, soon closed his eyes and had a sneaky 40 winks.

But as with any kid, there was a feeling that was much worse than boredom, and I was about to have my first taste of it: acute embarrassment. With the first test done and my cables detached from the machine, we were instructed to go off and get some lunch, before returning for some more tests in the afternoon. It was summer, I recall, and with no facilities on the premises, Dad decided the best thing would be to go and get something to eat at the pub on the nearby square and, as the sun was shining, to sit outside. Which was all well and good, except that with my bunch of cables – temporarily bound and now neatly taped to my shoulder – I still looked like something from a science fiction movie. And a scary one, if the stares I attracted were anything to go by, which seems a bit harsh, in hindsight, considering they were probably all nurses and doctors and must have been used to such sights. My humiliation only subsided when I saw another boy walk by and noticed that he had the same bunch of cables glued to his head. Had we been older, perhaps we would have shared a sympathetic exchange of nods. As it was, I could only count myself the lucky one, because he had it worse: he was in a dressing gown as well.

But not all my experiences of hospital were negative. While most of them involved pain, stress or ritual humiliation, sometimes they were actually very joyful. By the time I was 16 my brother Mark was into motorbikes, as were his mates, and when I was an inmate in the hospital for some more tedious tests a while later, a bunch of them decided to come and visit me. I was up on the second floor, but even so, you could hear them arriving before you could see them and the sound of them parking was fantastic, just like a fusillade. I looked out and there they all were, leather clad and looking impossibly cool. I couldn't have been more thrilled to see them.

Even nicer was the reaction of the nurses and other patients, when they saw the six young men in biker gear striding down the ward. No one could say anything, of course, but their faces were a picture. When they all left – having been perfectly polite, and not outstaying their welcome – I rushed to the window again, to see them roar off as one. I felt so proud, and so subversive, that I thought I'd burst.

16 February 2012

Breaking news: The jigsaw has landed!

Though, to be honest, it's not the one we'd originally planned on doing. The original, as per my list, was a whopping 5,000-piece job, which we'd borrowed from our friend June Pereira. It was a fine art image, which came with the rather grand title of *The Archduke Leopold Wilhelm in his Picture Gallery in Brussels*. It looked complicated – which, in jigsaw-land, actually made it easier: the more complex the picture in terms of shapes and tones and colour, the less likely it is to drive you to insanity. It's the seascapes and landscapes that really vex the committed jigsaw fanatic, which I am not. So it was a no-brainer in that sense.

But I could tell right away that it was going to be impossible: not because it was too hard, even if Ellie found it a little fusty, but because I hadn't factored in the sheer size of it. It was enormous! Not only would it not fit on the designated coffee table; it wouldn't fit on the dining table, either, and that was assuming that we'd be happy – which Lisa obviously wasn't – to have the table out of commission till the thing was finished.

In the end, Ellie and I opted for a 1,000-piece puzzle: a montage of famous steam engines (the *Flying Scotsman* and the *Mallard*, among others) which we think Lisa might have bought me years ago and which, as yet unopened, was gathering dust and cobwebs in the loft. And though it was no closer than poor old Leopold to her favoured subject areas of One Direction, One Direction and … let me see now … One Direction, Ellie pronounced it an acceptable replacement.

Doing the jigsaw is one of my more specifically CMT-targeted challenges; and not just for me but for Ellie, too. With CMT it's not just the lower limb muscle groups that are affected. It attacks the muscles of the arms and hands as well. This obviously has enormous implications for dexterity, and for both Ellie and me muscle wastage, and the accompanying loss of strength, mean our fingers can't do the things most people take for granted, such as unscrewing bottle tops or lifting heavy items like saucepans, or even something as simple as picking up something off the floor after losing grip on it. For me, with decades of practice at trying to find solutions, it's all about maintaining independence. Not being able to tie my own laces or put socks on or do up my top shirt button are all things that I have grown to accept are going to be beyond me on some days, because the weakness varies enormously day to day. But I've found solutions – electric can opener, electric jar opener, button doer-upper. Sometimes I just work out different ways to do things without any adaptations or devices. It definitely helps focus the mind on what I *can* do.

For Ellie, though, just starting out on the same journey, the challenges are still exactly that: challenging. We are incredibly lucky in that her school makes every effort to include her in all activities, but she still has to find ways of doing what others can and she can't. Her dexterity, though better than mine, is already causing her problems, and she's on the road, just as I was, of having to come to terms with the inevitable: that it'll be a process of continual deterioration. She is already having to learn to do all her writing on a keyboard – something that's perhaps not such a problem as it was back in my day, as kids these days, after all, are so competent with computers – but, as with so many things that she can't do but the rest of her peer group take for granted, it obviously marks her out, and that frustrates her.

As will this jigsaw, I don't doubt! It'll frustrate us both. And it's meant to, since it relies on the ability to pick up really tiny pieces and then slot them into very precise places. Daunting, but, as I hope to prove to Ellie, still achievable. It will just take time and commitment and lots of patience, and at the end of it, boy, will we both feel proud.

But even if we don't – even if, in the end, it defeats us – Ellie will still have learned a very valuable lesson: that it's all about giving things a go, having a stab at them. That's the key to having an exciting and experience-filled life.

Tonight being a Sunday night we decide to get stuck into it, while Lisa is in the kitchen ironing school clothes for Monday morning and Matt and Amy are occupying themselves upstairs.

'Let's see who can find the most edges the quickest, shall we?' I challenge Ellie, as we sit down together on the floor by the coffee table.

I say 'sit' but that probably gives the wrong impression. What I actually have to do if I want to be anywhere lower than my wheelchair is 'transfer' from it – which all sounds very measured and controlled. Which, of course it is. What I like to call 'controlled falling'. So I whump down, and immediately see a tactical error: I'm going to have to do this every single time we work on it, since the coffee table is too low for me to do anything from my chair.

But so be it. It's either that or relocate back to the dining table, and now we've started … And, hey, it won't be for long.

It's already dark outside, the remaining snow a silvery carpet in the back garden, and sitting here with Ellie, the two of us working at a shared endeavour, feels exactly the right sort of thing to be doing. Something to keep us occupied for the few remaining weeks till spring comes along. And I don't doubt, looking at the box, that it will take us all of that.

'Dad, *I* will, of course,' Ellie says with conviction.

And, since she's probably right, I'm not about to argue. Together we carefully pour the pieces into a heap in the centre, taking care not to let any spill onto the carpet, our dog, Berry (named by Ellie – being the youngest, she got her way there), not being fussy when it comes to unexpected potential food gifts. And yes, cardboard does fall into that category. I don't get much in the way of further conversation after that as Ellie, being Ellie, is too busy trying to beat me. In only minutes she's amassed an impressive pile in front of her – a pile that I notice is bigger than my own.

'There,' she says, as she pushes across a row of four she's already slotted together, niftily outranking the first corner piece I've just unearthed. 'Can we finish it tonight?' she adds, lining her handiwork up along her edge of the table. 'I bet we can, Dad. This is going to be so easy. Easy *peasy*.'

'That would be great,' I agree. 'But I think it might take a *little* bit longer.'

Around three weeks, I decide. Three weeks, tops.

* * *

As my condition progressed, so did the wastage of the muscles that had prevented my toes from straightening out as a little boy. So much so that by the time I was eight or nine, I was constantly falling over.

There's nothing positive about falling over, ever. Though it often made for unexpected entertainment for my classmates, for me it soon became the bane of my existence, as there was never any warning about when I'd next keel over. One minute I'd be walking along happily and the next I'd be flat on my face – literally. There was hardly a day that went by without my sustaining some sort of injury – usually a fat lip or a bloody knee.

I hit the dirt so many times in my formative years that it's a miracle, looking back, that I'm not a criss-cross of ageing scars, with a nose like that of a battle-hardened prize-fighter. As it is, I got lucky, because my nose is still intact – or perhaps it was the copious application of Germolene and ice packs and plasters that saved me. I only have to get a whiff of that pungent pink ointment to be transported straight back to my primary school playground; to the feel of grit embedded in my palm, the tears welling in my eyes and the suppressed giggles of my mates, who couldn't stop themselves. The girls, on the other hand, being more sympathetic creatures, would gasp in shock at what had happened, and disapproval, while some teacher or other ran to the rescue.

The reason for this sudden increase in falls was a condition I'd now developed called bilateral foot drop. If you can imagine losing all the muscles that surround your feet and ankles, the resultant floppy appendages – which they'd be, should you try to flap them around a little – will give you an idea of just how infuriating my feet had become. And once a foot doesn't do what it's supposed to – i.e. adopt the angle you tell it to – falling over becomes the easiest thing in the world.

But if my pride was wounded by having become someone who could no longer walk properly, that was nothing compared to the alternative I was given: a set of orthotic boots and calipers.

Most kids who grew up in the 1960s will remember calipers, mostly because at that time polio was still a significant problem in the UK. By the beginning of the decade, of course, vaccination had become widespread, but almost everyone knew one kid who clanked around in calipers as a result of having contracted the disease. (I always recall the first time I saw Ian Dury, perhaps the most famous musician of the modern era to be afflicted by polio. I remember thinking two things: what a brilliant bunch of pop songs he'd written, and how did he stop his calipers from squeaking?)

Calipers are designed to support the lower leg, and back then they consisted of a heavy, orthotic ankle boot (which looked very much like the kind of footwear Frankenstein's monster favoured, on account of its thick sole and bulbous, rounded toe cap), which contained a pin in the heel that connected to a pair of twin steel posts that ran up either side of the leg. These were attached at the top to a leather strap that sat just beneath the knee and could be adjusted to sit snugly around the calf. At the base of the steel bars there was a spring mechanism. This was what would allow my feet to extend, while at the same time, when I lifted my foot from the floor, pulling it back up to prevent foot drop and, therefore, all my falls.

Despite being made to measure, the orthotic boots – which came in black and brown (which was at least one more colour than Henry Ford offered, I suppose) – were extremely uncomfortable. And once fitted up with the calipers (they weren't the easiest thing to get on and off, either) even more so. Yes, they did their job – they kept my feet at right angles and prevented them from doing the dirty on me – but they also made me walk with a curious, Woodentops-style, stiff-legged gait; so while my older brothers were buying all sorts of trendy footwear in town, I had to endure the indignity of spending my time – in school and out of it – looking like Frankenstein's monster. At least from the knees down; from the knees up I tried to compensate madly, by adopting a winning smile. Though, given the discomfort, this was probably more of a grimace.

From the day that I donned those boots and calipers I felt different. I was suddenly, and irreversibly, conspicuous. Yes, I could walk around now without fear of falling flat on my face, but with the ugly footwear, the creaky calipers, and the steel bars that fitted attractively to the back of the boots, I now realized that I wasn't like any other child I knew. While the falls were just a part of me – and, let's face it, all kids fall over sometimes, some of them often – there was nothing else about me that made me seem any different to any other kid. But now there was. The boots singled me out.

It saddens me now, thinking back to my young self. I was so keen to fit in, so anxious not to let it get to me. But it did. How could it not? Suddenly – and it really did feel as if it happened the very day I first had to don them – my new legwear meant I became a pitiable individual. I was now the boy who was always picked last for a team in football. If I was picked at all, that is, for my ears began ringing with new phrases: 'Sorry, you can't play our game because you're not quick enough,' 'Sorry, we've got enough now,' 'Sorry, we need someone who can kick a ball straight.'

So off I'd trot, trying not to let the hurt I felt show, trying to pretend I had better things to do anyway, trying not to let it get to me. But it did, and my mother could see that all too well. My 'don't care' carapace wasn't thick enough for me to hide under – not with her.

'You know what?' she said one day when she picked me up from school, 'I was in town earlier, and I was looking in C&A, and they have some really nice new trousers in stock. Very modern.'

And she took me, right away, back into town so that I could try some on. She was right. They were very much the look of the moment, sporting, as they did, the widest flares imaginable. And crucially, as well as being achingly cool, they were wide enough to almost completely hide my calipers. I have a lot to thank the early 1970s fashion extravagances for, I guess. And even more to thank my mum for. I'll never forget that.

But even though the flares help to boost my flagging self-esteem, now I was in calipers I was officially disabled. No, there wasn't any official announcement, or formal piece of paper, but there didn't need to be. As any disabled person will undoubtedly tell you, once you become disabled, people begin to treat you so differently.

Which I suppose is understandable, but even as a child I remember finding it so frustrating that there seemed to be some sort of unspoken perception that the calipers on my legs had somehow affected my brain. That overnight I had suddenly become stupider.

Academically, I had never been at the top of the class, but neither had I been at the bottom. Yet now some teachers (not all: there were some notable exceptions) began to patronize me in a way that was completely unexpected. It was as though I'd broken both my legs and been fitted with a brace of plaster casts, and from now on it was their duty to protect me; to prevent me from doing something that could injure me further. It felt horrible. At a stroke it was as if I'd lost my independence. No, in fact it was worse than that: I *had* lost my independence, because they would no longer let me do all the things I used to do, despite being just as physically able – actually, more so – as I'd been before I'd had to wear the boots. They were my badge of office: the signifier that I was officially disabled, and needed treating as a disabled person.

Not that I wallowed in feeling aggrieved by all this, any more than I wallowed in self-pity. I had my moments of frustration, but I tried to make the best of it; perhaps on a subconscious level I was trying to be defiant. They might think I was disabled, but I would show them!

And my refusal to be sidelined seemed to hit home eventually. By the end of that year I think my calipers were less visible; though teachers would still hover nervously around me, perhaps the absence of a regular need for Germolene had calmed them and they felt able to relax a little more.

In any event, I was deemed fit enough to take on my first acting role – in the school nativity play. It was a progressively comic one and I was pleased to land a role that would demonstrate my talents in this area. It wasn't a big part – I had just the one line to rehearse – but it was one that was guaranteed to get laughs. Being good at headstands, I'd been hand-picked and my job was to deliver the line 'What's in this bucket?' and then fall forward and do a headstand inside it.

There was to be only one performance, so there was no room for error, and I took my responsibility correspondingly seriously. And I came good, saying my line loud and proud before doing the headstand, to a delighted whoop from a clearly impressed audience. The only thing was that in rehearsals the bucket had been placed centre stage, whereas on the night it was placed at the back of the stage, up against the wall, home to the school's highly polished set of wooden slats. Up I went – bash! – and down I came again, perturbed. Up I went again – bash, rattle! – and once again, down. Finally, the third time, I decided to stay put, my lower legs, as I tried to balance, drumming out a military tattoo, while the other children tried to perform their own lines over the din. When I finally came down – after however many noisy minutes with my shins rattling against them – the wooden slats that had long been the caretaker's prized equipment were so scratched and battered by my calipers that they looked as though they'd been set about by a man with a serious grudge. By the time I left the school they still hadn't had them replaced. Perhaps they are still there. I'd like to think so.

By the age of ten, fatigue had become an issue. I had always had a little trouble walking to and from infant school, and when I went to the juniors, though I walked around while there, my parents began to push me to school and back in an adult buggy. The thinking was that if I didn't tire myself out on the journeys, I would be less tired both while in school and when I got home.

Though not as big a thing as the calipers, the buggy ride to school was still an issue, as it made me an obvious target for bullies. Most of the time I did my best to ignore them. I had no choice. If I went after the bullies in school, I'd only fall over, which would naturally encourage them even more. Luckily,

I had a good friend – with whom I am still in touch today – called Andrew Russell, who helped me out of scrapes quite a few times. But there was one boy who was my nemesis. He was fast and he was mean and he was stronger than I was, and since I had spent so long falling over and knew exactly how much it hurt, I didn't want to be pushed over by him. In fact, 'didn't want' is perhaps understating my feelings about this boy: I could never get away from him quickly enough, and I would feel physically sick if I was in a situation where I knew it would be impossible to avoid him – not to mention his equally nasty sidekick.

Most of the name-calling I attracted was unimaginative and predictable – cripple-features, stick legs and so on. But one taunt was worse than others: spindle legs. 'There goes spindle legs!' they'd yell, whenever I came into view, and there was something about that one, particularly, that really upset me. I don't know why, but the picture it evoked really hurt.

Looking back it seems the easiest thing in the world to shrug such a taunt off, but at the time, as any child who's been bullied knows, it eats away at you, particularly if your self-esteem's already fragile because of standing out in the way that I did. It's a feeling I'm glad I remember in some ways, because it reminds me how far society has travelled in the interim. There will always be bullies, of course, and they will always find victims, but things are so much better, in that regard, for Ellie. Not only does she attend schools (specialist in the morning and mainstream in the afternoon) where she receives physio, support and all the help she needs to thrive, but there is also much wider acceptance of people with disabilities.

I was lucky, though, in that, like Ellie, I had brilliantly supportive siblings. Mark was in high school, of course, and Gary soon went to join him, but while he was still in primary school he always looked out for me. Though our paths didn't generally cross during the school day, he'd always make sure he was there beside me at going-home time, to tell anyone who dared bully me to back off.

But my best support was Nicola, my little sister. She may have been small but she was feisty and was my number one protector. Mess with me and you messed with her – and she was a force to be reckoned with. Still is.

Me and Nicola.

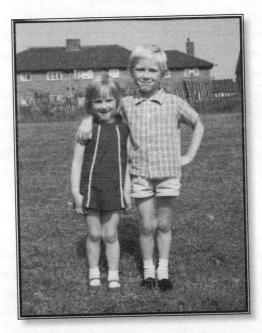

Which is not to say I was a pitiable figure in school – quite the contrary. Once I got to junior school, I increased in confidence daily. By then, I think I'd learned to play to my strengths, one of which was being in the right place at the right time, which suddenly stood me in good stead on the football field. I couldn't easily run after the ball, so I would goal-hang instead, and if the ball came my way I would just kick it wildly, in the hope that it might hit the spot. And the first time it did, there was a sea change in how my peers viewed me. No longer was I Mr Last-pick when teams were chosen.

I was also treated differently by the teachers once I hit junior school: while they still stopped me from doing things I felt perfectly able to do, they didn't seem to patronize me as much. Quite the contrary, in some cases, which was probably vital to my development; it wouldn't have done me any favours to become someone who thought he could get away with not doing things he didn't want to do, after all.

And I did my fair share of transgressing, like any other kid. A favourite transgression was not going straight inside after the bell had rung for the end of playtime, the punishment for which was having to stand on a black spot. I don't know who thought up this particular punishment, but it was a sound one, in that it was so public. There were six black floor tiles, altogether measuring about 20 inches square, which formed a pattern underneath the main school staircase. If you were naughty, you would be made to go and stand on one of these – a kind of 20th-century equivalent, I guess, of committing an act of treason and having your head stuck on a pole, for all to see, on London Bridge.

But standing anywhere for long was an issue for me. Though the calipers corrected my foot drop, they did nothing to aid my balance, so remaining stationary was a challenge. So it was odds on, I reckoned, that when a passing teacher noticed my plight, I'd be excused an extended spell in position. But it wasn't to be.

'Here we are,' she said, grabbing a chair from down the corridor. 'Sit on that.'

It was probably a useful life lesson, that one.

Another was more gradual but equally enlightening: how the world views you when you're long out of nappies but are still wheeled to school by your mother. Being in my adult buggy was an eye-opener from day one: a window on the world I would take my place in as an adult – a world that would see the wheels and treat me differently. I remember being pushed home by my mother one afternoon, and how the mother of a friend of mine stopped to speak to her. My father was unwell at that time, and had been home from work, so when the lady, looking concerned, asked Mum, 'How is he today?' we both naturally assumed she was talking about Dad.

'Oh, he's *much* better, thank you,' Mum replied.

It was only then, as the woman looked solicitously at me, that we realized she actually meant me. I was old enough to speak, intelligent enough to speak and, to cap it all, her son's school friend, yet because I was being wheeled home in a giant buggy, she assumed the correct approach was to talk *about* me rather than *to* me.

Looking back, I wish I'd mumbled and drooled all over her shoes.

But my time in mainstream school was fast coming to an end anyway. In 1974, when I was 12, it was decided I should be moved. Not to the local high school my brothers now attended, but to a state school called Martindale, in Hounslow, west London, which would be more suited to my needs.

Though a part of me really wanted to join my brothers at Harlington Secondary, in retrospect it would probably have been a nightmare. It had a lot of stairs, for one thing, and was quite a bus ride away, and having got there I don't doubt I would have encountered as many bullies as I'd left behind in primary school.

I was also, at that time, beginning to experience a marked deterioration in my hands, which was starting to make it difficult to write. Mum and Dad had recently procured a manual typewriter for me, and I was beginning to learn how to complete my written work on that. Going to Harlington, therefore, would have meant not only bus rides and stairs and bullies but also the prospect of having to haul a heavy old-fashioned typewriter around to every classroom in the school – like some sort of roving correspondent. No, on balance, Martindale School it had to be. And, despite it being daunting to go somewhere so outside my experience, I remember actually being quite excited.

My last day in primary school was mid-term for some reason, and for all the challenges I'd faced in coming to terms with my disability, my overwhelming sense – then and to this day – was that the vast majority of people were – and are – friendly and supportive. The friendships I'd formed there would give me the confidence to face whatever was next. My friends also gave me a leaving present to remember them by: a Timex watch, which the whole class had clubbed together to buy for me. I was so overwhelmed that it was one of only a few times in my life when I couldn't physically get any words out.

How I hope Ellie is similarly blessed.

23 February 2012

Mantra for the day: Lights! Camera! 50 List action!
Prayer for the day: Don't prang the Porsche.

6.00 a.m.

Everything to do with filming begins early. Everyone knows that. And I'm glad we all got an early night last night, because *The One Show* is no exception. Happily, it's half-term, so the whole family can get involved. And as half-term days out go, I am definitely the current hero; days out don't come better than this.

We kick off at 7.15 a.m. at a place called Airkix in Milton Keynes, where we've driven, as instructed, to meet the film crew.

'Will they actually say "action!" do you think?' Amy wants to know, as we pull up and get out to greet them.

None of us knows, but we're hopeful. It's certainly an impressive start. We're met by the producer, Matt Ralph, the presenter, Lucy Seigle, as well as a research assistant (the one with all the notes and itineraries, presumably) and a runner, who I assume does any required running. (It's all a bit manic, and to my shame – perhaps because the nerves have kicked in now – I don't get either of their names. So, belatedly, apologies and thank you!)

Greetings over, it's time to get the day properly underway and film the first of today's challenges: indoor skydiving. I have to keep pinching myself – I'm actually doing all these amazing things today! As I have been a thrill-seeker all my life, this is just about the best day out I can imagine, and I'm so grateful that *The One Show* has picked up on why I'm doing The 50 List: to show Ellie that if you really want to do something, then you shouldn't let anything stand in your way – little inconveniences like CMT included.

They've opened Airkix specially early (the power of Auntie Beeb, I guess) so that we can film before the day gets going properly and they can get their shots in the can – I'm already conversant with the correct lingo – without too many people wandering around.

Numbers have swelled now; we're also met by a cameraman and soundman. And once we're all assembled, the runner immediately runs off to find some breakfast. She soon returns with an array of egg, bacon and sausage rolls. They smell delectable, but given what I'm going to be doing before long, I barely touch mine. Don't want to bring it all back up again!

7.30 a.m.

Since Ellie's been invited to try the skydiving too, she gets to sit in on our short pre-flight briefing. This seems to clinch it: despite her initial enthusiasm, the combination of cameras and sound booms and safety rules and jumpsuits conspires to make her change her mind – she'll just watch. Which is fine. This is not about cajoling her to do things she doesn't want to but just to let her know that, if she does want to do, she can. Which she might well do some day, if not this day, after watching me having a go at it.

With me all kitted out in my flight suit, it's time for my first interview with Lucy.

'So, Nigel,' she says, 'why has this made your list?'

Not for the chance to dress up like a superannuated Superman, obviously. 'It's a bit of a cliché,' I tell her, 'but you're free as a bird up there. I'm out of my wheelchair. I'm not on my legs …'

Which, as I say it, reminds me what an incredible feeling that will be. I know I'm not on my legs anyway – well, except when I'm in a swimming pool – but to be free of gravity for a few moments, to be supported by nothing but the airflow, for there to be no difference between what the instructor can do and what I can do – well, *wow*, just the thought of that is so liberating. I still feel nervous. But I know it's in a good way.

8.10 a.m.

What a rush! The experience is incredible, as exhilarating as it is surreal. Basically, we 'fly' in a vertical wind tunnel, essentially a Perspex-bound room within a room. Once you're shut in it, the sense that it's a tunnel is even stronger; it has a mesh floor, below which is a 20-foot drop to the bottom. It's down there that the 'wind' that will lift us is generated, in the form of a large chamber that will expel airflow at approximately 140 mph, while above us is another 30 feet or so of headroom.

And the windflow – the air that will keep me aloft – is greater than any storm I've ever experienced.

It feels amazing. I say 'fly' but what I'm really doing, once my instructor pulls me into position and we begin spinning upwards, is falling at terminal velocity. That's the fastest speed at which a body can fall through the air towards the ground. Of course, I'm never going to hit the ground; that's the point of the upward draught. Because the air is pushing me upwards I'm 'falling' for what feels like minutes at a time, my cheeks being moulded so that I feel as though I have a rubber face. It's a powerful force; so much so that I have to wear goggles – without them my eyes would dry up like prunes. It's also incredibly loud, despite the ear plugs I've been given. It really is an assault on all my senses.

We come back down to earth, but in my head, I'm still floating. I can see Ellie outside, sitting on the viewing bench with Lisa, Matt and Amy. And I can see from my older two children's faces that they would both *so* love to be me right now. I make a mental note: must find the time and the money to allow them to experience this for themselves. Not to mention Ellie, even though I can see she has no appetite for it – not right now, anyway. Her expression is as anxious as Matt's and Amy's are awed. But though I know it has scared her, seeing her dad whirling high above her head in thin air, I really hope one day she tries this for herself.

Time to move on, though, and let someone else have a go. I can see a gaggle of new people now waiting, crammed into the flight room, all of them presumably thrill seekers just like me. Climbing back up into my wheelchair, I count around ten of them, and as I manoeuvre up to the seat I can't resist it. 'Brace yourselves,' I quip, as they look on, in some confusion. 'I didn't need this thing before I went in there ...'

12.30 p.m.

Arrive at Silverstone racetrack for the second of the challenges. The kids are in an ebullient mood.

'They said "action!"' says Matt. 'They actually *do* that. Go "action!" How cool is that?'

We all agree it's pretty cool. Also cool is Lucy Seigle, I privately decide. She is full of life and energy, clearly knows a thing or two about cars, and seems genuinely interested when I tell her about my lifetime of doing motorsport activities. She's also quite a character and, leading the convoy on the journey here, really put her foot down at one point. Needless to say, it was non-negotiable that I kept up with her. Rather a lot of male pride at stake ...

Once again the BBC team couldn't be nicer. I couldn't be more excited now that we're at a racetrack (I always am; in terms of earthly delights, it's my spiritual home, this) and also now that we're so close to another real highlight: being given free rein at the controls of a £60,000 off-roader, on their Porsche Driving Experience circuit.

It's been a good while since I've been able to do anything like this and I really miss it. My last off-road experience was something like eight years ago, when I was still able to walk a few steps. My then neighbour, Graham, had a 1985 Range Rover, which he bought to use on green lanes and compete in. He kindly made some small adaptations so that I could drive it too, and we spent many happy times swapping duties as driver and navigator when we competed in various off-road trials. But, of course, the thing about CMT is that it progresses all the time, so, even with the adaptations he'd made to make driving off road possible for me, my days doing it were always numbered. Which was why it was now high on my 50 List.

Incredibly, technology has moved on so much that I am going to need no adaptations to drive this intelligent, gizmo-stuffed 21st-century brute, and I can't wait to get going. My only regret is that the family can't climb aboard and do it too.

'Oh, but they can,' Matt Ralph tells me as we finish off our briefing with Jeremy Palmer, the instructor. 'Not with you, but they can certainly go out on the course with Jeremy afterwards.' He turns to Lisa. 'Would you like to?' he asks her.

I don't need to hear Lisa's answer to know what it will be. I only have to look at my son's expression. If mine's an 'icing on the cake' one, his is a 'cat that's got the cream' one. Cheshire cat as well, looking at that grin.

The Porsche Driving Experience circuit has been purpose built to demonstrate the off-road ability of their big 4x4, the Cayenne, and it's designed to take the car to its limits. It has a hill with a precipitious 1:1 gradient, side tilts – like skate-boarding ramps, only for grown-ups – that will force you to drive at a 45-degree angle, ascents and descents with the same sort of slope, and a section of course with a surface that's so uneven that you mostly have to drive over it on two wheels.

In short, for a bloke like me, it is heaven. As I navigate it, half my mind is on how pleased I am that the kids will get a turn on it too. Matt especially. I half relish and half fret at the realization that he might have inherited my thrill-seeker gene. He is, I know, really going to love this.

And he's not alone. Once I'm done and out of the vehicle (which, incidentally, now looks much like a horse that's just finished a steeplechase – splattered with mud and lightly steaming), I'm almost bowled over by the stampede of children (not to mention my previously dignified and patient wife) all intent on being the first one to get in.

'Whoah!' I command, as Mattie calls shotgun on the front seat and claims it. I'm conscious that Matt Ralph still has to get a second tranche of sound bites, but it's like trying to stop a tide by putting a hand out. No one seems to mind, anyway – who wouldn't be raring to give it a whirl? Though seeing their grins of excitement – Lisa's too, it must be said – I find myself smiling. From where they were waiting for me, they couldn't see even the first part of the course and they have *no idea* what they have let themselves in for.

Matt is first out of the car when they return to base 20 minutes later. While they've been on the course I've been rootling around the Porsche showroom. They have a few Porsche GT cars – the ones they use for racing. Oh, how I'd love the chance to try one …

Matt leaps down from the Cayenne like a pro, his eyes wide.

'That was AMAZING,' he pronounces, before I can even open my mouth to ask him. He's a teenager, which means everything good is AMAZING – he deals in absolutes – but I can see this experience is even more AMAZING than most.

'Dad,' he goes on, 'the car almost fell over! Literally! It was, like, how could it possibly *not* fall on its side?!'

'I know,' I begin, nodding.

'And then we went up this hill. And it was this steep!' He levers an arm up, to demonstrate. 'And then we're the other side, at the top, and then he took his foot off the brake, and, like, it was AMAZING! The car didn't even *move*!'

'I know,' I begin again. 'The one in one hill, ri –'

'And then we went across this other hill, and the car was almost *sideways*!'

'And it was *brilliant*!' chimes in Amy, who has just come and joined us. Like her brother, she is ball of pure excitement.

'You enjoyed it, then?' I ask them, though the question feels unnecessary, and I feel a sudden and intense moment of happiness. It means so much to me to be able to share such moments with my children, and particularly important where Matt is concerned, because he's a boy and I want him to feel he can have as good a time with me as all his friends can with their dads.

'Dad,' Matt says again, perhaps reading my thoughts even as I think them. '*Enjoy* it? It was AMAZING!'

But it seems not everyone's quite so enamoured of the off-road experience. Namely Ellie, who has an expression that speaks volumes. It says: 'Humph! Who was it who talked me into *that* nonsense?'

'Not for you, then?' I ask her. I can see it might even have frightened her. She's a little pale, I notice, and clinging on to Lisa's hand – something I imagine she probably did for the duration.

'No,' she said. 'It wasn't. I couldn't even sit in my seat properly. I just kept sliding around all over the place. And it was scary.'

Which is a salutary lesson for me to keep in mind as I do this. I might want Ellie to *think* like me, in terms of how she approaches life with CMT, but I still have to remember that she *isn't* me. Not everyone sees adrenaline in the same way as I do, after all, or feels my drive to create a level playing field for myself, so that I can enjoy the same sense of achievement everyone else can. Then something else hits me: would I have liked to be a helpless passenger, being chucked around in the back, out of control? Put it like that and I suddenly get it. Emphatically not. Perhaps we're not so different after all.

1.00 p.m.

It's already been a long day, but it's not over yet. We've now travelled south, to a watersports lake next to Thorpe Park, where I'm going to do the last of my extreme challenges of the day: drive a powerboat – another thing I've been itching to try my hand at.

I've never driven a powerboat before, but I have been on the water, having been a member, for a time, of the British Disabled Water Ski Association around 15 years ago. It was great fun – I water-skied behind some pretty fast powerboats back then – but since I fell off my water-skis almost as often as I stayed on them, I never got the chance to feel the thrill of speed on the water; I was too busy feeling the cold and the indignity of being repeatedly dunked in the drink.

71

The boat I was hoping to drive today (but can't for pesky health and safety reasons) is another brute, in terms of power. It's a ski boat with a huge V8 engine, and as a passenger, I know the instruction I'm going to need to take most heed of is also the simplest: 'Hang on!'

So I do hang on but, even so, as we launch, hard and fast, I'm gobsmacked by how quickly we get moving. It feels like seconds – correction, it *is* only seconds – before we've reached the other side of the lake. The boat comes to a stop and as I wipe spray from my eyes, my instructor, James, grins at the look of awe on my face.

'Quick enough for you?' he wants to know, as we swing the boat around for the return trip. Drenched and speechless, I can only drip and nod. *Wow!*

But the fun's not over. As we begin making our way back towards the jetty James turns abruptly (can he sense that I'm a speed junkie?) and we're off again, speeding across the water. So I'm doubly wet by the time we pick up Matt Ralph and the soundman, who are this time coming too, so that they can shoot some more footage of the experience from on board – principally of my reaction to the launch.

In fact it's not my reaction to speeding off that's most arresting. As we launch again, the soundman, who's chosen to sit on the engine cover, very nearly falls backwards into the lake. So that's it. My response to being in that huge V8 power-boat? Not wow, or OMG, or anything excitable, as you might expect. It's fits of laughter. But no matter: it's in the can.

8.30 p.m.

Wow! What a day!

And what a long day, as well. Unsurprisingly, being full of so much adrenaline, I was still buzzing when we parted company with Lucy and the team, but when, ten minutes into our drive home, I glanced across to speak to Lisa, it was to see that the whole family were sound asleep. Which was no surprise either: we were up pre-dawn, after all, and it felt (still feels) as though we didn't stop for a second. The kids even got to have their own go in the powerboat. Which is perhaps – I sniff the air as I drive the last couple of miles to home – why the windows are steamed up and the car smells so distinctly of pondlife.

I'm tired as well by the time we're home, but not nearly as tired as Ellie. I know the day, for all its highlights, has exhausted her. Not too much, I hope. I want her to take only positives from it, and to keep it stored in the back of her mind for times when she faces her own challenges, as both Lisa and I know she will. I want it there as a reminder whenever life gets frustrating, which we both know is going to happen, too. I want her to think to herself: *Look what Dad managed to do, despite his CMT. And if he can, then I can* ... That's what I hope. Even if it doesn't mean getting behind the controls of a 4x4. Which it won't.

'Did you enjoy yourself today?' I ask her, as Lisa gets her a glass of milk. She's in her pyjamas. It's way past her usual bedtime. She must be shattered. She nods, rather than answers. I think she's too tired to engage. 'What was the best bit?' I prompt her.

She thinks for a second, and I'm expecting something along the lines of 'When you did this ...' or 'The part where you did that ...'

It's not. Me doing stuff is not on her mind, clearly. 'Um ... What was that thing?' she wants to know. 'That thing they kept shoving up your jumper?'

'That was a microphone,' I explain. 'They put it on me so that they could record my voice. Without it they wouldn't have been able to hear what I was saying.'

Ellie takes her milk from Lisa and sips it while she takes this in.

'And what was that big fluffy thing on a stick they kept holding?'

'That was a microphone too,' I say. 'Just a bigger one, that's all. A boom mike, I think they call it.'

'Because it makes your voice boom?'

'No,' I tell her, chuckling. Though I'll concede it's a logical enough thing to wonder. 'The "boom" bit refers to the long pole they dangle it from. You remember that? So that it can hang down where everyone's talking.'

She drains her milk. 'Ah,' she says, taking this in as well. 'So that they can hear everyone talking at once?'

Now I'm floundering. I know almost nothing about audio – a lack Ellie seems determined to expose.

'Erm ...' I begin, but she's already yawning, so instead of trying to come up with answers I kiss her goodnight. 'Sleep tight,' I say. 'Another early start in the morning. More jigsaw puzzle to get done, eh?'

She nods again. It's only when she's halfway up the stairs

that she remembers my original question. 'The best bit was the boat,' she says. 'Being splashed is really fun.'

Which I think is probably good enough for me.

24 February 2012

Number of challenges now completed: 3 of them. Finally. Can't thank the BBC enough.

Number of jigsaw pieces finally in place: Numerous. We have the whole edge done now. Just that not-at-all-daunting-huge-gaping-hole in the middle and we're done …

10.00 a.m.

I could get used to this. As if yesterday didn't hold enough thrills and spills for one lifetime, today, yet again, Ellie and I are to be in the limelight, as another film crew will be turning up on the doorstep any minute now to get some footage of us in our natural habitat, doing normal things together, which will flag up for the viewers just how CMT can affect people's lives. Obviously, being wheelchair-bound has already been covered in my various challenges, so in this film they want to concentrate on the less obvious ways CMT can affect quality of life.

One of the most challenging aspects, as I've already mentioned, is lack of hand dexterity – using a knife and fork, aspects of getting dressed, opening tins with a tin-opener and so on, and, for me at any rate, the frustration of dropping money on the floor and it being nigh on impossible to pick it up again (I keep my wallet on a very tight leash). Ellie's hands are still reasonably strong, and though she has a tremor, it doesn't affect her, but watching us together will, we hope, show the viewers the bigger picture – the reality she might have to face once she's my age. So we're going to do things like operate the remote control, turn on power switches, tie some shoes laces and also add a few pieces to the jigsaw, all of which will demonstrate lack of dexterity and raise the profile of CMT generally.

It's not showbiz, of course, but, *yes*, I think, as Ellie makes her final sartorial decisions, *I could definitely get used to all this.*

7.30 p.m.

Actually, perhaps not. I am clearly not a natural on TV.

Although as being a TV star was never on my wish list – now or at any time – that's not important. This has been all about raising awareness of CMT, and in that sense, I've done what I set out to.

They were a team of just two today – a soundman and a cameraman. They arrived at around ten this morning and got busy. I'm a semi-professional photographer myself – I've had a few pictures and reports published in the local paper, and I am technical editor of the online magazine *Drag Racing Confidential* – so I was immediately interested in all the kit they brought with them. When you see stuff on TV, it all looks so natural, but in reality there's a whole array of technology that helps them achieve that. Key among this is a small but incredibly complex lighting system, which can achieve lots of different tones of colour – and, best of all, without daubing anyone in orange face paint.

The filming itself took around half an hour, most of which was centred on the jigsaw (yup, the dreaded jigsaw). On this occasion, though I had Ellie to help me, we weren't graced by added 'help' from Berry, as the soundman was allergic to dogs.

And I was clever. Before we filmed, I removed half a dozen of the pieces that we'd already put in place and strategically located them as if we hadn't, as one of the great realities of doing a big jigsaw is that first you have to *find* a piece, and when you're still at the 10 per cent stage (i.e. you still have 900 in the box – gulp) – well, the team could have still been waiting there ten days later.

That done, and the other agreed examples of dexterity issues in the can, it was time for me to do my 'piece to camera'. The idea of this was that one of them would pose questions out of shot, which I would answer looking at the lens rather than them. *This is good*, I thought, remembering my fundraising efforts; *now I have a chance to really connect with the viewing public*, and other self-congratulatory things like that.

Then, before we knew it, they were gone again, keen to rush back to BBC Television Centre in London, to get the whole thing ready for the piece to be shown on television that very night.

'You know what?' I said to Lisa, as we convened on the doorstep to wave them off, 'I am a bag of nerves. Who'd have thought it?'

'You'll be fine,' she said.

It was a tense afternoon, even so. Had I said the right thing? The wrong thing? Had I talked absolute rubbish? Had I inadvertently – horror of horrors – picked my nose? Probably not (it's not a habit I engage in, I hasten to add), but when you know something you've done is going to be seen by over four and a half million people, it tends to make you quake just a little.

In the end, as it turns out, it was fine.

'That all looked rather good, I thought.' Lisa was first to comment. She was right. The piece having been condensed down to however many minutes, my main impression was one of speed. Not just my own speed – through the air, over the water, doing, ahem, the jigsaw – but that my 15 minutes of fame still has some time in reserve. Blink and – bar that shot of me in the boat, laughing my socks off – Nigel Holland, suave TV man, was gone.

But, boy, was it fun, and boy, am I grateful. Only one minor omission hangs unspoken in the air, and I'm not going to be the one to point it out. Despite my quiet confidence, I was obviously talking absolute rubbish after all, because of my 'piece to camera' there was not a trace.

27 February 2012

Number of challenges completed: Er ... still only 3.
*But ... number of challenges started: Ooh, loads. Well, in my
    head, at least.*

Number of times I have passed the jigsaw puzzle and sighed:
  Well into the teens now.
Number of pieces the dog has eaten: Definitely 1 that we
  know of.

Today's challenge is the one on my 50 List that I've been looking forward to the most. But first, I am going to need to get a
grip. Literally.

The challenge is 'Play the drums' – something I haven't
done in a long time. I used to do it regularly and well, but now,
though the passion for percussion is still there, the grip isn't,
so I've had to resort to taking measures.

It's actually been a relatively easy challenge to organize. My
friend Clive has a superb Roland electronic drum kit, the
'kind' kind – one that doesn't annoy the neighbours. And with
a long roll of sticky bandage taping the drumsticks to my
hand, I'm all set. I can get reacquainted with flans, paradiddles
and super-imposed polyrhythmic patterns without the risk of
fatal injury via flying missile.

*   *   *

Forget appearances on TV and being the UK's only wheel
chair-bound drag racer (more of which later). It was as a
drummer that I probably had my finest hour, fame-wise, playing for a band called This Temple Eden. We were headed up
by a talented singer/songwriter called Darren Hill, who I met
at a music youth club. We started jamming together almost
straight away and around three months later met bass player
extraordinaire Phil Barker. Our first gig was at Hounslow Art

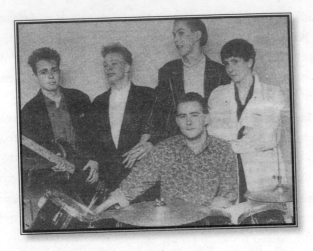

A promo shot for This Temple Eden. Look at the outfits!

College. We went through a number of names before we finally plumped for This Temple Eden, which was taken from one of Darren's compositions. He wrote some great songs, which I really enjoyed drumming along to, and he is still hard at it. Today he's working as a freelancer writing Christian resource material. The final line-up also included Gary Holder, guitarist, and Ian Gray, playing the keyboard.

This Temple Eden gigged at venues all around London in the 1980s, including the Clarendon in Hammersmith and the Academy Rooms at Brunel University. But our Greatest Gig Ever (I can hear the kids saying 'Yes, Dad, we *know* ...' even as I type this) was an appearance at the Leicester Square Hippodrome, though when I recall it I tend to brush over some of the finer details. It was during *Children in Need*, and we were due to play our set right after some audience participation on stage. I was as excited as I'd ever been about playing anywhere – this was the big league! – and even more excited to be playing somewhere posh enough to have a proper drum riser below the stage, from which I would rise, like Neptune from the waves.

Having done a brilliant sound check earlier, we were all pretty psyched up by the time we were suited and booted and I had to go to my drum kit under the stage. The deal was that I'd wait there till the stage manager pushed a button, and as my band mates strode onto the stage from the wings, I'd be elevated into position with my drums.

To my horror, that wasn't what happened. The button was pushed and right away I could tell things weren't right, because the sounds from above didn't seem to fit. There had been no announcement, no cheer – either for whoever was departing from the stage, or arriving on it – and as soon as I cleared the surface, I could see why: I was rising up behind a tableau I'll remember till I die – of the then Radio 1 DJ of the moment, Gary Davis, busy with some clippers, shaving some man's head for charity.

They cleared the stage eventually and, once they'd managed to stop laughing long enough to come and join me, my band members arrived and we played what we thought was a pretty blinding set, even if it was quite a culture shock for the audience. But I will never forget how much of a prize plonk I felt, sitting in the middle of the stage, marooned and blushing scarlet, while Gary Davis calmly razored someone's bonce.

Attaining such a dizzy height of fame was no flash in the pan. My passion for music had begun early. While my lower legs and feet had given me all kinds of grief throughout my childhood, my arms and hands had worked pretty normally. And like any other child, I had a favourite way of making music. For some this might be the recorder, for others the flute, but for me it was always the drums.

It was an interest that began developing in earnest in my early teens, just after I went to Martindale School. I had a love of music generally, and would spend hours listening to my records. I loved rock, particularly Pink Floyd, Rod Argent, Supertramp, David Bowie and Led Zeppelin – any band that had a solid rhythm section, really. And as I listened I was always focusing on what the drummer was up to. It became something that was almost instinctive.

Initially, my 'drum kit' was of the basic variety, a few upside-down biscuit tins and a couple of my mum's knitting needles, but eventually I was able to progress to the real thing, as there was a youth club in Uxbridge, run by the local youth service, which started up a twice-weekly music club called Feedback. It was like a temple to cool, at least to my untutored eye: a place where young wannabes could indulge their love of music and satisfy their desires to try out real instruments, without completely deafening their parents.

By now, my fine motor skills were going. The muscle around the thumb was progressively getting weaker, causing me to have difficulty picking things up and, if I managed to do so, keeping hold of them. Having opposable thumbs is a really handy tool that the man upstairs designed for us: it's what separates us from all other species, and enabled *homo sapiens* to develop the use of tools, which is why not having them is such a bloody nuisance. But that was my lot, so learning different ways of going about doing things was pretty much all I could do.

But as with so much with CMT, at least I had some time to get used to it. It had begun with a loss of strength in my other digits – my fingers – and with my writing beginning more and more to resemble that of a doctor (or the progress of a drunken spider who'd stepped in a puddle of black ink). It was a wonder the teachers could read anything I wrote. It was about then, therefore, that I embraced the manual typewriter, and would inexpertly bash out my homework on that.

When I first started drumming I still had some strength left in both hands, which meant I could hold the drumsticks. But, frustratingly, it didn't last long. The muscle wastage gradually reduced my grip so dramatically that fixing the sticks to my hands with medical sticky tape was the only practical and workable solution.

I was happy to put up with it, just as long as I could play, because one play on a proper drum kit and I was hooked for life. It was as instant as that. Better than that, even, I clearly also had natural talent. 'You show real promise,' one of the club leaders commented when I'd finished. It was only as I began puffing myself up with pride that he added the damning caveat: 'Because you certainly can't get any worse!'

So that was me told. But ever the competitor, it didn't put me off – it spurred me on. I would learn to play the drums and learn quickly. I was keen to learn properly, too – from the experts. To this end I even travelled down to Croydon one weekend, so that I could attend a masterclass by my favourite drummer of them all, Billy Cobham, who was and still is a superlative session musician, together with the then drummer for Simple Minds, Mel Gaynor. They both played solos, answered questions and showed us a range of tricks and tips, and in doing so inspired every drummer in the room to do better.

Of course, talent's something you can't teach, and I will never have theirs. I always tried hard and worked hard, and I became competent enough, but I never really moved far on from thinking loud equals good; I never managed to master that musical sensitivity. But if I could just bottle their dedication, their exuberance and their ability to transmit that, and then give it to my own kids, I'd be happy.

29 February 2012

Number of challenges completed once today's is done: 5. Or a tenth. And still 9 months in which to do the other 45. So I am actually on target now. Hurrah!

However … number of friends who might decide to unfriend me by teatime: 1, if I'm not careful. Almost definitely.

Motto for the day: Skulls are delicate.

Feel like I'm on a roll now – in more ways than one. With the drumming ticked off, I'm on a different kind of roll: rolling the wheels of my wheelchair to pull some wheelies.

I'm not going to be alone doing it. I'm going to show someone else how to do it. When I put 'Teach someone to balance on two wheels in a wheelchair' on my list it was because it seemed such a great thing to be able to do that I wanted to share it. Not because I am some sort of deranged sadist, but because pulling wheelies in a wheelchair is a fundamental skill. Once you master it, you can go pretty much anywhere.

Which was why it occurred to me that it might be both entertaining and instructive to teach an able-bodied person how to do it. My friend Ian Blackett is not only able-bodied but also someone, like me, who enjoys a challenge. He's another speed freak, too, and also carries the distinction of being Santa Pod Raceway's official Run What Ya Brung photographer: as well as taking press photos, he provides a photographic service to racers who bring the cars to the strip to race them on public days. He was also instrumental in getting me my first press pass there back in 2005.

So I won't be mean to him. Before he arrives, I bring in my spare chair from the boot of the car, and before letting him loose on it, I let some air out of the tyres. With flatter tyres, the chair doesn't roll quite so easily, which will give him that vital bit of grip when he tries to pull his wheelies.

Even so (and to my secret relief, because I'm still just as competitive as I was as a teenager) it takes a few attempts and a couple of unplanned altercations with the sofa before Ian relaxes enough to remain static for a few seconds, even though his knuckles are white.

'This is much harder than it looks, isn't it?' he observes (somewhat stating the obvious, to my mind) as he hovers there, too terrified to move for fear of keeling over for a third time, while Lisa and his wife, Paula, make a sterling effort to suppress their giggles. He's lucky the kids are out playing, at least. But 'hovering anxiously' does not constitute 'confidently pulling wheelies'. The plan is that once he's mastered the art of static balancing on two wheels, he'll be able to do something useful with it – in this case, turn through 360 degrees.

Which is why all of this is taking place in the conservatory and not the living room. Can't have him keeling into my only nearly finished historic steam engine ...

* * *

Leaving mainstream education to move to Martindale, though slightly daunting, was very liberating.

And instantaneous. Armed with my box-fresh new Timex, and basking in the luxury of suddenly being allowed to wear anything I liked to school, I left the familiarity of my primary one day and started at my new high school the next. No time to get anxious. No time to prepare. No time even to think about it. Which, in hindsight, was probably the best way.

Martindale was a school for children and young adults with disabilities. Unlike my junior school, which was a pretty standard 1960s issue, it was built back in the late-Victorian era and even though it was fresh and clean indoors, you could tell it had its origins in a different time.

It had clearly been built with disability in mind: every wall in the place was painted white, down to a dado rail that was also a handrail so that those who had problems walking could hang on. The walls below the handrail were institutional red-glazed brick, and high above them, from the white-painted ceilings, hung lights that were suspended on chains.

The main corridor was also the main hall for the school, and it was here that we'd gather for morning assembly every day, as well as for lunch, and sometimes playtime, if it was raining. Off this vast space was a door to every office and classroom, the latter, on one side of the building, also having a door out into the playground. The floors were highly polished, the air still and faintly fusty, and the whole impression, when I first entered the place on a warm early summer morning, was of bigness and new challenges and growing up.

I think my parents were more anxious than I was that morning. Plucking me from my old school mid-term and depositing me in an unknown place, with unknown people, they must have felt nervous on my behalf about what lay ahead for me. I was nervous too, but instead of intense trepidation, as I might have expected, my overriding feeling was one of sudden freedom; I was no longer in a school that contained my nemesis, and that was enough to fill me with positivity.

It was a long journey to the school – a 5-mile slog through the heavy rush-hour traffic – and though any nerves had subsided by the time we arrived, I knew they'd be back with a vengeance once Mum and Dad had finally left me on my own there.

When we walked in through the swing doors that led into the big hall, Mr Higgon, the headmaster, was there to welcome me. He was a big man, in his late sixties, and stood with his hands clasped behind his back, his gaze unwaveringly on me as we approached him. He wore an itchy-looking suit made of a hairy checked material, and on his feet were very shiny brown shoes.

'Well, Nigel,' he said to me, once my parents had left. 'Here we are. Welcome to Martindale School.' His pride in the institution he oversaw was obvious. 'I'm sure you'll enjoy yourself here *enormously*,' he added.

His voice boomed in the huge space and, though his expression was friendly, I think I knew straight away that he wasn't someone to mess with. He was intimidating in the way those consultants the McArdle brothers had been, and I would soon learn that his background was the forces – flying Mosquitos in the RAF. I held him in the sort of awe that any boy at that time would. He was a leader, and had the respect of all the pupils because he'd served in the Second World War.

Mr Higgon took me personally to join my new class, and as we walked he asked the usual chatty questions. Had I enjoyed my time at my last school? Was I a little nervous about joining this one? How did I get here this morning – did my parents bring me on the bus?

Though I didn't as yet know of his background as an airman, I recall being inordinately proud to be able to tell him that my father, who'd brought us in the family car, was a driver at Heathrow, working for BEA.

I also marvelled, as we walked, at this completely new environment. I passed wheelchairs, pairs of crutches and walking frames, all parked neatly against the hall wall. There was even a red trike that you could pedal by using your arms, the like of which I'd never seen before.

Having arrived at the right door, Mr Higgon turned the handle and ushered me in to meet my teacher, Miss Jerome. I didn't know if she was married or not (I still don't) but she had the prim air of a schoolteacher you'd find in a storybook; she was a mix of sharp lines, stern looks and the odd flash of reassuring maternal warmth. I took the seat she pointed out to me, which was next to a boy called Andrew Skelton, who had Duchenne muscular dystrophy and was wheelchair bound.

Andrew and I made friends immediately, and later that same day we both played in a game of football, though it was the sort of football with which most people would be unfamiliar, given the disability and lack of mobility involved.

Andrew, playing in a wheelchair, opted to play in defence. This was a good move, because a wheelchair represents a formidable obstacle to get around, particularly if you're hampered by being unsteady on your feet. As I was, but at least I was still on them at this time, so I took my place up front for the opposing team. At that point (and, with hindsight, I admit somewhat at odds with the evidence) I rather fancied myself as a striker, so when I was selected to be penalty taker following an early foul by the other team, I was thrilled. I opted not to mention to my generous teammates that there was no telling where the ball might actually go.

I could kick a ball OK, but the trajectory was always something of a lottery, and since whoever had painted the goal posts on the playground wall must have had a goalkeeper as a cherished relative, the odds on my actually scoring a goal were, realistically, rather long.

Still, I was the new boy and my teammates were being kind, and I had a duty to do my best for them. I would at least give it my very best shot. While I was ruminating, however, the other team (who had objected to the penalty being given in the first place) staged a protest by putting every single one of their players in front of the goal.

Given that the odds of the ball ending up on target were so slim, this seemed like overkill, but I was determined to get it 'in' there if I could. Trouble was that with two wheelchairs and three walkers crammed in goal, the only area of exposed brickwork was the patch immediately above Andrew Skelton's head. So be it, I thought; then immediately I thought something else: that it wouldn't be much of a gesture of friendship to my new pal if, in scoring the penalty, I also took his head off. But to score a penalty on the first day in my new school would be brilliant.

I took aim, kicked the ball – or rather, as was my way, toe-punted it – goalwards, and, to my disbelief and delight I managed to hit the only exposed part of the wall. In doing so, I scored my first penalty and sealed my place as part of the team – and, I like to think, secured my fellow footballers' respect. Yes, it was so close to Andrew's head that it very nearly gave him a new parting, but somehow this went down as evidence of great skill. And I wasn't going to put them straight, was I?

Andrew and I remained friends throughout my time at Martindale, but sadly he died young, as people with that condition often do. It was in 1980, when I'd moved on to college. I'm sure he's much missed by everyone who knew him.

Martindale wasn't just a revelation in terms of what it had to offer me. It also opened my eyes to the disabled world. This was my first time in the presence of so many other disabled children and it was a little disconcerting, to say the least.

Unlike me when I started, most of the other boys were in wheelchairs, though one used crutches and one seemed to have absolutely nothing wrong with him – which led me, as anyone of that age would, I suppose, to speculate madly about what his disability could possibly be.

I was fascinated by everything, and very curious. We had a lesson that first morning, but for the life of me I couldn't tell you what it was, because I was much too busy checking out my new classmates. And they me, I don't doubt, so it was with a sense of mutual intrigue that we greeted the ringing of the bell.

We were lucky as ours was one of the classrooms that led out onto the playground, and once again I had a sense of being a kid in a sweetshop. Unlike the bland expanse of concrete that formed the playground at my junior school, this was a playground that really looked like a playground. There was so much to play with that I could hardly take it in. There were all sorts of different bikes, two sets of swings (normal ones and ones with harnesses) and even pedal carts. I was open-mouthed. Was this really a *school* playground?

As first days in new schools went, it was brilliant.

I settled in quickly. The environment was so welcoming that it would have been hard not to. I don't think I'd fully realized how liberating it would be not to be faced with stairs every day, for one thing; and as being here also separated me from my primary school bully and all his cronies, it meant my natural confidence could start to return.

Naturally, there was a bully to be found, though. And, as is inevitably the case when there's a new kid on the block, he (happily, there seemed to be only one of him) made it his business to find me. He was a big lad in a wheelchair – I think he also had Duchenne muscular dystrophy – who obviously tried hard to affect an intimidating air, but it fell rather flat because in reality (as I very soon found out) he had very little physical strength. In an effort, presumably, to make up for this lack, he had a misguided mate of his push him around the school, the better to let everyone else know who was boss.

When he decided it was time to put his marker down with me, I was sitting in the classroom one playtime, because it was raining, when I became aware of his wheelchair being pushed up alongside me. Looking back, it seems hilarious – him having to be manoeuvred into a position to bully me – but, nevertheless, that's what happened. And once wheeled into place, he brought his fist down, hard, on my thigh.

I had experienced bullies before, obviously, and my usual *modus operandi* had always been (sensibly) to avoid confrontation: don't let them get to you in the first place or, if they do, walk or run away. But this was different. He didn't scare me. He had nothing with which to scare me. Well, apart from his scowling henchman, who couldn't hurt a fly. So I held my ground. After all, I was both stronger than him and faster. I simply told him to back off and leave me alone. No way was I going to join the ranks of his tragic minions and spend my days pushing his wheelchair round the playground.

And to my great pride, he never bothered me again.

Perhaps the most important thing about Martindale, however, was that the school gave me my first self-propelled wheelchair. To say it was an exciting time is something of an understatement. It was one of the defining moments of my young life. Suddenly self-propellable, I regained my independence. It's hard to overstate what a big deal that was. Since just past toddlerhood my trajectory, in terms of independence, had been steadily downwards; as my condition deteriorated, so my dependence on other people had escalated. Now, at a stroke, that had been reversed.

It was such a revelation to realize, as soon as I started pushing the wheels, that there was virtually nowhere I couldn't go. It was so liberating to be free of the tedious business of having to lean against things, hold on to things, clutch at things in a panic, just trying to balance on two feet without falling over. It was so relaxing to be able to sit and engage in a conversation without half an eye on nearby supports and half my brain engaged in balancing – which obviously gave me a big boost in confidence. It was also liberating because suddenly I felt way less tired. Much as I'd previously wanted to cling on to the 'independence' of walking, being self-propelled – as opposed to the dependence of being pushed – made me feel free

And having a self-propelled wheelchair introduced a whole new box of delights: I got to join a wheelchair training class.

This confused me at first. I had a wheelchair and I knew how to push it. What on earth could 'wheelchair training' teach me that I didn't already know how to do? With my new accessory providing me with such a boost to my self-esteem, I had already wasted no time in training myself. I was quite the expert, starting and stopping on a sixpence and slaloming around people and objects like a pro.

But it turned out that I was in for a treat.

I was pulled out of class that first day by the school physiotherapist, who took me down to the physiotherapy department and told me the plan was that she was going to teach me how to pull wheelies. I was open-mouthed. Wheelies were stunts you did on push bikes – dangerous stunts. Something I knew from painful experience. Both my brothers could do them, and I'd always held them in awe, because for the brief time I owned a bike, I'd tried doing them as well, and found out the hard way that what looked so easy when Mark and Gary did it wasn't easy at all. Yes, I could lift my front wheel off the ground, just as they did, but no sooner had I done so than it reared up like a bucking bronco, flipping the bike over and me onto my backside. I think I managed no more than 1.2 seconds before it invariably went horribly wrong.

'*Really?*' I said, with typical 12-year-old excitement. I couldn't believe it. It wasn't just doing wheelies on bikes that adults tutted about; hadn't we always been ticked off in junior school for leaning back on our chairs as well? And here she was, telling me she was going to teach me to do just that. In a wheelchair, too. It sounded thrilling.

And it was. Though I hesitate to crow, I was obviously a natural, as it only took a short time to master the art of balancing on just the two rear wheels – a direct result, I suspect, of wanting to grab the opportunity to show that here was a wheelie I *could* do.

Not that this was seen as a party trick. As became evident once we started going out of school in our chairs, it was actually a vital skill to learn. The school was adapted to make wheelchair use simple; everywhere was flat or, at worst, had only the smallest incline, so getting around was a straightforward business. But out in the real world – the world that was overwhelmingly able bodied – pulling wheelies was the only way to manage.

It was fine to begin crossing a road – you'd just let your chair 'jump' off the kerb – but once you'd crossed it (observing the Green Cross Code at all times, of course) you were stuck: that 3 inches of kerb might just as well have been a 6-foot brick wall. But once you could do wheelies – i.e. lean back and balance your big wheels, so lifting the front two smaller ones – you could get the front wheels into a position where they rested up on the pavement, after which all you had to do was pull up yourself and your chair.

It obviously took arm strength, which, fortunately, I still had; thankfully CMT doesn't affect the muscles of the upper arms. And I helped to build up my general fitness in the process, which stood me in good stead in lots of ways.

Learning to do wheelies at the age of 12 had one other big effect on me: it was probably the genesis of what would become a lifelong competitive streak. Which was something the school was obviously keen to foster. And as a consequence, all thoughts of 'disability' melted away. With so many of us in wheelchairs, being seated felt perfectly normal; and, like any other school, we had a full programme of sports activities – they were just different ones: we'd regularly compete with each other in wheelchair races and giant slaloms, and I found I had an aptitude I would never have even known about had I remained in mainstream education.

Best of all, I won regularly; I still have the gold medals to prove it. Between 1972 and 1976 I regularly won golds for both wheelchair slalom and the 60-metre-dash wheelchair race. I even had the honour of representing Martindale as part of our team for the national school games at Stoke Mandeville, which was one of those occasions when I didn't mind that I didn't win a medal. Yes, I'd have liked to, but I was just so honoured to have taken part in what would go on to become the Paralympic Games.

Sport was a big part of my life at Martindale. As well as the wheelchair racing I joined the archery team and again managed to pick up some gold medals. I was so passionate about it that Mum and Dad even bought me my own bow and arrows – at great expense – so that I could compete outside school as well. I remember how awful I felt when there was a fire in the archery club one night, and my bow and arrows were destroyed along with everything else.

Trying everything was something of a philosophy at Martindale, which, as an adolescent full of energy, really suited me. As well as archery, I tried discus and shot put. But my favourite field sport was javelin, and I also loved competitive swimming: two more disciplines that bagged me gold medals.

In all this one thing was a constant, and it was a constant that probably shaped me: finally I was in a place where no one would think of shaking their heads and saying, 'No, Nigel, I don't think you can do that.'

At Martindale, for the first time, I felt I could do anything. Though I was soon to find out that wasn't true.

MARCH

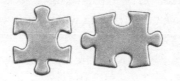

4 March 2012

Big exciting news!
Number of leading figures in the world of steam locomotion
  currently in possession of all their faculties: A big fat 1.
  Well, not that big or fat, to be fair. But nevertheless a
  striking chap. Stove-pipe hat. Groovy yellow waistcoat.
  Name of Isambard Kingdom Brunel.

He is marooned in space, though. He and a small section of his impressively detailed blueprint. Which is what happens with jigsaws. You make progress in increments, creating lots of little islands of connected jigsaw pieces – islands that are destined to an extended spell of homelessness, being shuffled around a central abyss of coffee table to suit your needs. Often neglected (once you're tired of looking for that elusive 'purple piece with a bit of white on it'), they sit marooned while the edges of their universe come together with such agonizing slowness that before it comes to pass, Stephen Hawking could probably have written a chapter about the phenomenon for a whole new book.

Safe to say, I am beginning to hate this jigsaw. This jigsaw I am working on, sweating over, picking up piece by errant piece, which, all too often, I have to retrieve from the dog. We're only a few weeks in, I know, but I have had a small epiphany. The completion of it is going to be very, very hard.

'I hate this jigsaw,' I tell Ellie as we sit together on the floor doing it. Matt and Amy have become canny now – and so soon in the process. They see me sitting there, they see the box of pieces on my lap, they flee.

Not only that but their friends flee as well. Yes, they look at it, and might even venture to comment on its progress. But actually do any of it? Well, of course not. They are much too polite. This is my and Ellie's challenge, so it wouldn't be seemly. Guys, just *do* some! No one need ever know …

Poor Ellie. Does she rue the day?

'You don't hate it,' she tells me. Confidently. 'You say you do, but you don't really. Anyway, it's exercise for your fingers.'

She plops a piece into place, which will allow a small lump to join a bigger lump. Which abuts the Great Western Railway logo on the far left. I keep ploughing through the box, looking for a purple bit with some white on. Which, for all I know, might now reside inside the dog. It's the not knowing that's so hard.

To be honest, it's a miracle we're sitting here at all. Well, not the sitting bit so much; rather the fact that the jigsaw is still here in one piece. Mattie had some mates round last night and when I came down this morning, our living room resembled not so much a living room as the underside of a flyover – the sort you find in big, edgy cities. No smoking braziers or help-ful souls handing out leaflets about homeless shelters, but in most other respects, you could have stumbled into one of those earnest documentaries that shed a light on the dark underbelly of society. Sleeping bags everywhere (some of distinctly dubious provenance; there was one there that I distinctly recall seeing gathering cobwebs in the garage recently); mismatched duvets and pillows strewn all over the carpet; empty 2-litre Coke bottles; wizened curves of discarded pizza crust; nuggets of toffee popcorn clinging to the sides of an enormous bowl.

Actually, scrub that last bit. You probably wouldn't find toffee popcorn under a flyover. But you might – given that the vagrants would quite possibly be bored with being vagrants – have expected to see some progress on the jigsaw: it's just *there*, after all. Or (and I expect this would have been more likely, what with teenage boys being teenage boys) to find it in more pieces than before.

But neither happened. Hey ho. On we go …

*   *   *

Though I had made friends at Martindale, we were all fairly scattered, the nearest friend living over a mile away, and most of them around six miles distant. So at weekends, at least for the first couple of years, I still met up with my friends from my old school.

And now I was a little older, I was keen to experience a bit more freedom – something that had been lacking at my junior school.

I'd had a bike back then, but only very briefly, and because it wasn't a very good one it was difficult to ride, and useless for pulling wheelies. So instead I had to fall back on the only means of transport available, the adult buggy, which someone obviously had to push me around in. Now, though, I had gone up in the world, because the disability service had delivered me my first adult trike. It was nothing special; painted blue, and very functional, it didn't lend itself well to being customized. Even at that age, seeing my mates adding spokeys and stickers to their push bikes, I could see that accessorizing mine similarly might mark me out as a bit sad. I wasn't stupid. I knew no amount of tinkering with the aesthetics was ever going to make it – or me – look cool. It was suggested that it might be helpful to have a basket fitted to the frame behind me, but I resisted. If there was one thing I didn't want it was a basket, and particularly there. The fact that I could give lifts to mates gave me a bit of credibility – and I wasn't losing that for a frigging basket!

For all its design disappointments, though, the trike was brilliant. It had three gears, so coped well with at least minor inclines, and it meant I could escape the house and start going where my able-bodied friends did – which, at the age of 12, meant pretty much anywhere I wanted. It was never that far – to one of my friends' houses, or to hang out at the local playing field – but, again, it represented real freedom.

And, naturally, now I had my new wheelie skills to work with, it wasn't long before I was pulling crazy stunts on the trike too, lifting the left wheel up in the air so that I could ride it like a normal bike. In truth, this wasn't just for the sake of showing off, although it was another thing that gave me a bit of credibility. Trikes couldn't go to lots of places where bikes could, being so much wider, so if I wanted to stick with my mates I needed to learn how to get through all sorts of barriers. Which felt quite thrilling, once I'd properly mastered the art – a bit like 007, in one of the Bond movies, where he tips a Mustang on one side so that he can use it to chase the villain through a narrow alleyway.

Not that James Bond had my share of irritations to contend with. Sometimes, though I'd done nothing to deserve it, I'd be grounded, stuck at home and trike-less, for the simple reason that my dad, who did some night shifts, was in bed, fast asleep, having parked his car in the way of the shed where it was stored. To wake him up and ask him to move it would, of course, be unthinkable. On those occasions I would have to make do with my self-propelled wheelchair, which was better than nothing, but unless you're an elite athlete, keeping up with a moving bike is impossible, and I was lucky to have such brilliant, patient mates.

The wheelchair also attracted the sort of attention that no self-respecting adolescent boy wants. It was hard to look cool when some well-meaning adult came along and just grabbed the rear handles (in those days, self-propelled wheelchairs often also had these) in the misguided belief that I couldn't get by on my own. At such times, being a polite boy in the main, I'd try to be gracious. But every so often I'd get really shirty. I remember one poor man, keen to help propel me down the pavement, getting a real tongue lashing from me.

'It's OK,' I began (nicely). 'I can push OK myself, thanks.'

'No, it's fine,' he replied. 'I don't mind pushing you.'

Which obviously triggered a burst of waspish teenage fury. 'How would *you* feel?' I railed at the poor man, in high dudgeon. 'How would you feel if I got hold of each of your legs and started trying to move them for you? *Well?*'

I think I even finished off by saying, 'Don't touch my chair again!' But though I cringe to think of it, I also feel sorry for my young self, for my sense of self-esteem was as fragile as any other boy's, which meant that developing some independence, limited though it might have been, was important. I was growing up in a world that wasn't quite geared up for me, and I needed to know the limits of what I could and couldn't do.

Which meant, as well as batting away offers of help now and then, pushing the boundaries. And sometimes further than my mum would perhaps have wanted, which was why, sometimes, it was best that she didn't know.

My friend Paul Cawthorne and I would often go into Hayes on a Saturday, to spend what little pocket money we had. Paul was my mate, and had been since we were both about five or six. We hadn't become friends in the most likely circumstances. We'd met at the local swimming pool and, as Paul well remembers (yes, I have his emailed confession), I was the little lad sitting at the side of the pool who he decided to push in. It was nothing personal; just something he decided to do for a laugh, having had it done so many times to him. Of course, he didn't know I had a 'disability' – how could he? – and he was promptly thrown out of the pool. This apparently upset me (the details are hazy; my memory's more amnesic goldfish than Paul's is) but it seems that I didn't want this potential friend to disappear, and as a result, while he was drying off in the changing room, crying his eyes out, the pool attendant told him he could stay after all.

Our friendship was a match made in heaven. Well, kind of. Because we got into all sorts of unholy scrapes. Most notable was the time when my dad had just spent hours fixing my broken wheelchair (the result of some ridiculous stunt I'd done), only for Paul to give me my usual tow behind his bike the same day and for me to crash, breaking it all over again.

We camped out that night, the pair of us, in a tent in Paul's garden. It was cold, I remember, but anything was better than facing my dad that afternoon.

At the age of 12, money always burned a hole in our pockets, so finding something to buy with it was a regular occurrence, be it chocolate, cans of Top Deck shandy or new records. But it wasn't just the shopping that we enjoyed; it was also the trip to town, because our route took us over a busy main road bridge that ran over the railway lines that led into central London. There was a steep incline up to the middle of the bridge, and a similarly precipitous one the other side, so the reward for the big push to get the wheelchair to the middle was a chance to properly road test the chair's capabilities, or – to use language that any 12-year-old boy would understand better – to see how fast it would go.

Looking back, when I see the bridge now I'm faintly appalled at our recklessness. And we *were* reckless. To further test it, we'd both ride the chair, bombing down the pavement, with me on the seat and Paul clinging on behind me, his feet on the pegs at the rear, till one of two things happened. Either we'd come to a stop, my hands burning, as I gripped the wheel rims to slow it; or, as happened on one memorable occasion, I'd make an error with the steering, which on that day changed our trajectory and resulted in an altercation with a tree. Luckily, I was thrown before my head hit the trunk and, though we both sustained a few bruises and bumps and scratches, it is the pain in my stomach from laughing so much that remains my abiding memory of the occasion.

Like any teenager, I suppose, I would have my down times. There were always going to be moments when I'd rail against my disability; days when some frustration or other reminded me of what I couldn't do, and I'd have to speak to myself pretty sternly. I'd been brought up to be positive and keep focused on my blessings, and, because I'd had my condition since I was too small to recall the start of it, I had by and large adapted to each small deterioration as it came along. Feeling sorry for myself wasn't something I had to actively avoid doing; it simply never occurred to me to do so.

But one day, when I was 14, things took a sudden nosedive I stopped being able to run.

I suppose I had probably been lulled into a false sense of security. I'd been at Martindale School for two years now, and life there felt normal. And, crucially, nothing much had changed. There had been no real deterioration in my condition to adapt to, and if I didn't actively worry about future deterioration, it was mostly because it didn't much figure in my thinking; I lived day to day and most days felt the same.

It wasn't as if I was running a great deal, because I got about in school mostly in my self-propelled wheelchair. It was important to do so in order to preserve my energy. There was also the constant issue of making an unscheduled acquaintance with the stone floor – something I was keen to avoid. But I still liked playing football and would regularly risk my nose for it; out on the school field landing was that much softer. I also enjoyed joining in for the odd session of rugby, where falling over, traditionally, was part of the game anyway, and where I did have the odd minor tumble. (Not that tumbles were to be desired. With so many of us either in chairs or unsteady on our feet, the school would have had to have a shuttle to A&E permanently at the ready if we'd played the game the way the able-bodied played it. So Mr Knight, who taught us geography but was also an ex-player, devised a version that used intercepts rather than tackling.)

But one morning – or what felt like one morning, anyway – I woke up and found I couldn't run any more. In reality, the disease had been progressing continuously, the muscle wastage that is one of the key features of CMT creeping up my legs to my knees and thighs. But whether or not I was in denial about how bad it was getting, it seemed that one day I could run and the next day I couldn't.

It happened so suddenly. I had always accepted that running would gradually get harder; I knew that bit by bit I'd play all the various sports just a little less. But I have no memory of a gradual realization that the business of running was getting tougher. On this day, in late summer, it was as though a switch had been flicked – a watershed moment. I tried to run, and suddenly I just couldn't.

Both physically and emotionally, it devastated me.

It was on a school day, in the playground, when I realized what had happened. I saw the ball rolling across the tarmac – an invitation to anyone who wanted to play – and as I started to run towards it, it seemed that the lower part of my legs was dragging; it was a real effort to bring each leg forward quickly enough. It's as difficult to describe as it was to comprehend. I continued to try to run, but then I fell over.

I picked myself up, caught my breath, brushed the grit from my knees and palms, and tried to struggle on, attempting to play as I'd always done. But it was so hard, and in the end I decided I'd better be goalie; valuing my nose and teeth, I decided it might be safer.

But that too was harder than it had ever been before, and I could think of little else for the rest of the day. Why were my knees feeling so weak? Had I damaged them and not realized? I thought not and, little by little, a more depressing truth emerged. This might be it. I might just have reached a stage in my condition where the muscle wastage had reached a crucial point; I might never be able to run again.

Running is something most people probably hardly think about, but when you do think about it, it's central to being human. Though most of us will hardly ever need to use our fight-or-flight reflex, it's still the key thing a person can do to get themselves out of trouble, help someone *in extremis* or get something they need for themselves.

I was not going to need to run after my dinner, obviously, but not being able to do that one thing felt bigger than any other. It wasn't just the functional issue; it was the sheer exhilaration that came with running. Despite my acceptance of the freedoms being in a wheelchair had brought me, losing my ability to run made me feel wretched.

And angry. I came home from school on the coach that day seething with frustration and anger. For the first time in my life, I said, 'Why me?'

It must have hit me harder even than I initially realized, for as soon as I got home and told Mum what had happened, I found I could hardly get the words out to explain it to her. Instead, I broke down, which, because I'd always been so accepting and pragmatic, I think really shocked her. It was as though a floodgate had been opened, which washed away the carapace I'd been carefully building all that day. I had never felt anger at my condition like this before – anger *and* frustration – and it hurt.

'But why me?' I kept saying to her, over and over. 'Why did I have to have this? Why not someone else?'

Mum had no answers, obviously. How could she? She and Dad must have been as bewildered and upset about it as I was; they had probably felt the same distress as soon as I was diagnosed. They had had to deal with the reality, every bit as much as I had, that I would not only not get better but also get worse. It must have been so hard for her, so painful to have to witness – something I only fully understand now I have Ellie.

So all she could do was comfort me, as I raged and cried at the kitchen table, and accept my shouts and accusations – she had given birth to me, after all – and wait for the storm to subside a bit.

Later on that night, after tea, when I was calm enough to listen, Mum and Dad tried to sit me down to talk about it properly. But I was still much too upset to sit down and be talked to.

'You know, son,' said Dad, sitting down himself, beside Mum, 'the trick is how you think about it, really.'

I didn't know what he was getting at, and said so. I had what I had, didn't I? How was mere thinking going to change this wretched curse I was saddled with?

'You're wrong,' he argued. 'How you think about a problem can change everything. Making the best of things invariably makes everything better.'

I still couldn't see that. 'How?' I asked. 'How will thinking anything make things better?'

'Because it will make you concentrate on what you *can* do,' he explained patiently. 'It's the only way to approach life. If you want to get on and make something of yours, at any rate. Course, you *can* feel sorry for yourself – and everyone does sometimes, that's only human – but where will it get you to wallow in self-pity all the time? What will it help you to achieve?'

'I know that,' I argued irritably. 'I get told that all the time in school.'

'But there's a difference between knowing something and actively embracing it. Running isn't everything, Nigel.'

I knew that as well. But right then, not being able to do it felt as though it meant my life was over. Running *was* something that meant everything to me.

'But it's not everything,' Dad persisted. 'It feels that way at the moment, but not being able to run isn't the only thing in the world, you know – it doesn't mean that there aren't other things you can do.' This time he didn't give me a chance to say 'I know ...' again. 'Look,' he said, pointing to the wheelchair I was refusing to sit in, and which was parked – as if to taunt me – in the corner of the room. 'How many kids do you know who can do the tricks you can do in that thing? Hardly any, I'll bet – *including* your mates at school. You can do them because you put in the hours practising – and that's the key to it. And how many people', he went on, 'do you know who've competed in archery competitions as you have, who have medals for it, hmm?'

He was right, of course. Hardly any.

'And how about your racing?' He pointed towards the wheelchair once again. 'How many people have got the medals you have for slalom racing?'

Ditto.

'So you see,' he said, 'there's so much you can do that others can't. Running is just one thing. Not everything.'

Dad patted the chair beside him, and now I did sit down. 'Don't let this one thing colour everything,' he counselled. 'Instead, take it on the chin and don't let it get to you. That's the best thing you can do, you know – look yourself squarely in the eye and think: *Oh well, so I can't do it this way any more. I'll just have to see if I can do it a different way.* That's how everything gets done, you know – how everything's invented. By humans doing what they do best.' He tapped his head. 'By thinking around the problem. And finding solutions. Do you see?'

I nodded. Because, finally, I did.

Or was beginning to, at least. And it was probably after that day and that conversation that I worked out my own personal mantra: to take things on the chin and approach every problem life and CMT threw at me with one conviction – that if I couldn't do something one way, I would simply, by trial and error, find another way to do it instead. I would adapt. Because adapting was the most important thing I could do. If I didn't, I would no longer be someone with a disability. Instead, I would be something I didn't want to be, in my head or anywhere else: a disabled person.

6 March 2012

Number of challenges completed: 5, not forgetting that respected 19th-century civil engineer.
Number of days before the Silverstone half marathon: 5.

Brilliant. Just brilliant. Less than a week to go until the half marathon, and – how infuriating is this? – I have a cold.

I tried to blame the kids, obviously, because that's what you do. And given that I'm being so stoical and not referring to it as flu (of the man kind or otherwise), I was hoping for a little more sympathy. I also have a cough, which is potentially more disabling, as when I cough I struggle to breathe more than most people do, as I have only one working vocal cord.

This was something that didn't happen till I was 40, which was probably why it never occurred to me, when I started getting odd symptoms, that it was anything to do with my CMT. As anyone else would, when I was hoarse while talking on the phone to a friend one morning, I assumed it must be some kind of virus. But it was odd, because although I sounded as though I had a very sore throat, my throat wasn't actually sore at all. And the hoarseness seemed to take ages to go away.

When it came back, it returned with a vengeance. I was at church one Sunday, chatting to the group of youngsters I took for youth group – or rather trying to – when it began giving me serious problems. This time I had been suffering from a cold for a couple of weeks previously, and was at that annoying stage when you get a dry, tickly cough. Talking to the kids – about not making decisions based solely on first impressions, I remember – I kept having to clear my throat, as the tickle just wouldn't seem to go away.

I was mid-cough when it happened: all of a sudden I couldn't breathe. Try as I might, I could only get the tiniest bit of air into my lungs; and the more I began to panic at the alarming rasping sound my throat was making, the worse my breathing got. I could tell there was some sort of obstruction in my windpipe – that I was choking – so I gestured to one of the teenagers to go for help.

They returned with the best person they could have, Trisha Gilyead. She's a nurse and was able to assess things in an instant, though her conclusion – call an ambulance as a matter of urgency – was perhaps not the best news I could have heard.

Being unable to breathe properly has always been something I've been afraid of. No doubt everyone feels the same. One thing's a constant: when I leave this world I don't want it to be from lack of oxygen. It wasn't surprising, then, that I went into panic mode quite quickly – certainly as soon as it became clear that, despite my coughing, whatever was choking me wasn't clearing. And panic is the last thing you want in such a situation. The more I fought to breathe, the harder it became *to* breathe, so, though I was clearly getting sufficient air (I'd have passed out if not; I knew that) breathing was a real act of will, and I didn't know how long I could keep it up.

Thankfully, the ambulance didn't take too long to arrive, and within seconds of being assessed I had an oxygen tank beside me and a mask, on which I sucked very, very gratefully.

Once at the hospital I was taken to the high-dependency unit, where the oxygen, the machinery and the presence of so many medical professionals combined to ease my anxiety sufficiently for me to breathe less shallowly, and we could actually talk about what might be wrong with me. Once I'd explained how it had started, an ENT consultant was whistled up, and it was decided, though I was clearly in no immediate danger, to keep me in hospital for a couple of days to conduct some tests. I might have baulked at this – tests being the bane of my life – but it's amazing how thinking you might have fetched up at death's door tends to concentrate the mind.

The following day the consultant arranged for me to have my nose and throat scoped. This was a necessary evil to get to the bottom of the problem. Despite anaesthetic spray, it really is the most unpleasant sensation, particularly if the sinuses are blocked. It became clear why the problem had arisen: one of my vocal cords was relaxed and not working. This was a mystery that obviously needed further investigation. At the same time, to help reduce the inflammation caused by the cold, I was put on a course of steroids and antibiotics.

A few days later I returned to the hospital, and after further inspection, was told that I needed to have a scan. I can't remember the type of scan: CT, MRI, Star Trek Tricorder, who knows? I only remember it being big enough for me to fit in, just. By this time I was feeling more relaxed about everything. Perhaps this was just some weird CMT symptom, which the scan – giving a much clearer picture of what was happening – would be able to clarify. So when the result came back 'negative' it took a little while for me to twig. It was only my mum's reaction – one of joy – that really hammered it home for me: they'd been looking for (and perhaps expecting there to be) a growth that might have been pushing on one of the nerves that worked the vocal cord. Looking, as Lisa pointed out, for a tumour.

As it was, I was just unlucky with my personal experience of CMT. Vocal cord paralysis, as I subsequently found out, can be one of the many possible symptoms, but it's also an extremely rare one – I've only once come across another CMT sufferer who has it (ironically, it's the current chair of the CMT organization). If I were the type to feel hard done by, I guess I would.

I was down for a good while after that episode; to lose the strong voice I once had was hard to come to terms with. And though I tried not to dwell on it, I was also very frightened. If one vocal cord had just stopped working out of the blue, how long before the other one gave up on me – and what then? The thought of losing my voice completely was a scary one. Not just from the point of view of becoming mute, either: with two vocal cords flapping about I knew that breathing could become a serious issue.

But so far, so good. And I suppose I must count myself lucky: I got away with it for 40 years, so things could have been worse, and day to day it isn't that much of a problem. Yes, I do sound a bit Barry-White-crooning-at-the-ladies when I have a bad cold and get episodes of stridor, but unless I get a bad one I can live with it easily enough. So whenever surgeons have suggested a laryngectomy (removal of both my vocal cords) or a tracheostomy (an incision in the windpipe to make a direct airway), just to be on the safe side, my answering no doesn't involve any deliberation. I can face losing lots of things, but my voice isn't one I want to contemplate right now. As the kids would probably tell you, I like the sound of it too much!

11 March 2012

Number of challenges that will have been completed once today is done: 6.
Mind you, number of miles to be completed around Silverstone racetrack today: 13.1. (And yes, that .1 does matter.)

6.30 a.m.

I'm not going to let on to anyone, obviously, but I'm a bag of nerves this morning. So much so that I'm awake before Amy comes in, as she customarily does, bearing a wonderful cup of tea. She is a tea-maker *par excellence*, is our Amy.

Yes, *that* nervous. That's almost unheard of in our house. I'm hoping it's just all part of some big and ultimately useful adrenaline rush, but I feel slightly lightheaded at the thought of what I've taken on by doing this.

Still, an exploratory exhale and a tentative cough are reassuring. I still have the wretched head cold, and my chest has that bruised, constricted feeling that comes from night after night of coughing repeatedly (might also have been Lisa thumping me to get me to shut up, come to that) but as the doc has pronounced me fit-ish enough and well-ish enough to compete, that's it confirmed. No last-minute sick note. I'm competing.

The whole half-marathon idea was a curious one, really, because before I came up with the idea of doing The 50 List, it would have been the last thing I'd have thought of having a go at.

'Half marathon, perhaps, Nigel?'

'Don't mind if I do. Only one caveat – not in this lifetime.'

I never actually had that conversation, of course, but if someone had asked me, I'd have definitely ruled it out. Pushing myself and my wheelchair round 13 miles of race circuit just didn't float my boat. Because I was too hooked on manoeuvring much faster things round one, perhaps?

But when I wanted to include something on the list that would really test my endurance, it was almost the first thing to pop into my brain, right after 'Sitting through an entire episode of *Loose Women*', which would obviously have been too extreme, even for me. I wanted a heavyweight endurance challenge on the list, because dealing with something like CMT is all about endurance in so many ways; the day-to-day grind involves a great deal of it, because so many activities are much harder to achieve than they are for most people.

So this is a big one to set an example to Ellie, which is perhaps where the nerves really have their root. Gadding about in supercars and speedboats is one thing. This is another; this is pure slog, and I need to show her I can do it.

Of course I can do it. That's what I've been telling myself since I sent in the application. But there's only so far that sheer bloody-mindedness can take you. There's also the business of preparing your body for the task ahead, and in that, on the whole, I have scored a big fat zero. Yes, I've been trying to lose weight (one of the tasks marked 'other' on The 50 List) but 'try' has been very much the operative word. And that's even before I've attempted 'Make a crème brûlée' with its necessary taste-testing, so the outlook was always looking less 'aerodynamic' than 'airbag'.

My main concern since I sent the form in has been the weather. Yes, it's fine today, but it's felt like the worst winter in history – freezing cold, endless rain and then, to cap it all, feet upon feet of snow. Snow that was still lying around the garden till mid-February, which has meant that my training, since those first couple of tentative tours of Wellingborough, has been virtually a non-starter. Wheelchairs don't do snow; end of. (Note to self: possible new business opportunity to work on for *Dragons' Den*: invent snowplough attachment for same.) Then there was – is – the wretched cold, of course, which continues to be a pain.

But there's no point in sitting here running through all the possible excuses I'm going to be able to allow myself if I fail to finish the course. I *have* to finish it. Not getting round is not an option, and that's the end of it.

11.30 a.m.

It's obviously important to get to a race venue in good time (don't London marathon runners turn up about five hours beforehand or something equally crazy like that?), but it does nothing for the state of the nerves, believe me.

Though Lisa and the kids and I only got here about an hour and a half or so early, it already feels as though I've been here forever. I'm all checked in now, I have my race number, I have my timing chip. All I need is for the nerves to settle down sufficiently so that I can lose this unexpected development of feeling completely overwhelmed.

'You'll be fine,' Lisa reassures me as we all head down to the start, the kids all togged out in their CMT T-shirts, and Ellie clutching the sign she's made to wave, in order to cheer me on. But even though I know I'll probably *be* fine (I have to be; I want the kids to be proud of me), I don't *feel* fine; I still have the same tight chest and tickly cough.

As soon as I'm out on the track and get a sense of the scale of what I'm about to do, the feeling of being overwhelmed grows even stronger.

There are 17 wheelchair runners in the marathon today. I know because I've done my research. The most experienced of them race from the front, in their specialist racing wheelchairs. They have to; otherwise all the two-legged runners would get in their way. For they are *fast*. They are also pretty famous, in some cases; among their number is gold-medal-winning Paralympian David Weir, which is an inspiring thing to know in itself.

But people in wheelchairs like mine – in this context they are formally classed as 'day chairs' – run within the normal running mass. I'm in the middle of that mass now, and all I can see are torsos. Nothing else. Seeing torsos is fairly usual when you spend as much time as I do in a wheelchair, but in this environment, with so many of them massed around me, ready to race, I feel as a small child must when in the centre of a big crowd of adults, except without the reassuring mummy to hold my hand.

It's not just that I'm being a wimp; it's a real worry. My immediate thought is of safety. If I can't see anything beyond the person in front of me, can the people a couple of bodies behind me see me? Probably not. Which surely means there's a real risk of people running into the back of me and falling over me before they properly see me.

I glance to my right and see a woman who looks as though she might be a bit of a pro at this. She's a taut mass of colour-coordinated Lycra and toned body, and has a gismo strapped to her arm that I'd bet my last farthing is an MP3, heart monitor and GPS combined. I know this because I very nearly succumbed to buying one. I do love a gadget, me.

'Have you done this before?' I ask her, and she nods, removing an earbud from her ear so that she can hear better.

She's bouncing on the tips of her toes as she answers. 'Done a few,' she says, smiling, and I suspect she's actually into double figures. You don't get to look that fit by dabbling.

'This is my first,' I say proudly, and she nods again, beaming encouragement.

'Brilliant,' she answers. 'Good luck. Have a great time!' With the emphasis on the 'great', which I can't help but think is perhaps the wrong adjective to use. Still, I think, there are always endorphins in the equation. I just hope mine are standing to attention.

So as we get under way, that's what I decide to do: have a great time. When I get under way, that is. It's a good quarter of a mile before I even make it over the start line, during which I just move with the tide of people around me. But when we finally cross the marker, I move up a gear. Not Mach 1 – I'm not insane, and I'm still coughing and spluttering – but enough to blow away the last lingering shreds of anxiety and replace them with a cool breeze of air on my face and the inspirational sound of the cheering crowd.

Then I spot Lisa and the children – particularly Ellie, who looks so tiny compared to everyone and is frantically waving her sign, chanting the words written on it: 'Go, Nigel! Go!!!'

It does the trick. Now I'm properly fired up for the task ahead. All I have to do is keep doing this till I've gone 13 miles and I'm done.

The first 5 miles pass in a pleasing haze of motion. Yes, I'm hot – the weather's turned out much milder than I expected – and I'm having to drink water at every opportunity, grabbing a bottle at each water stop and stuffing it between my thighs, sipping intermittently so that I don't run out before the next stop. I'd intended to mark each completed mile with a jelly baby, but had to dump that idea as soon as it became obvious that jelly babies and dry tickly coughs are incompatible; the first has me spluttering like crazy.

I see no one else in a 'day chair' and it's a pretty weird business, being a lone wheelchair user in a sea of moving runners. I find that I pass some people and others pass me. I'm enjoying myself now, watching this sea of humanity in action. I could sit for hours in town people-watching, and this is no different, bar the fact that we are moving en masse. I'm fascinated by the diversity of the people running around me. Though united by a common goal, each individual has their own cause; with me it's CMT – and I think I'm the only one – but many charities are represented. There are people in crazy costumes, who must be sweating absolute buckets. I attract a few curious stares of my own and wonder why that is, until I twig that I am the only person on the whole race-track sporting jeans. And it feels so good – great, even – to be a part of this happy gathering, even if I'm momentarily disheartened to find myself overtaken by a speeding carrot at one point. I get him back: a mile later, and he's a root vegetable with issues; he bolted too soon. Now it's my turn to pass him.

Then disaster strikes. At mile six, I almost wreck my marathon. I don't know how it happens, because it's not as though I'm a rookie when it comes to pushing a wheelchair, but, perhaps in my haste to press on, I take my eye off the ball – well, the wheel rim. I manage to get the little finger of my left hand caught between the wheel and the actual rim, and almost pull the finger right out of its socket.

The pain is so intense that it almost brings tears to my eyes, tears not just of pain but of anger at myself, and I'm forced to slow down considerably for the next two dozen yards so that I can scan the side of the track for a medic. Perhaps I can have my little fingers taped to my ring fingers; it seems the only way of ensuring it doesn't happen again.

Finally I spot a medic and weave my way across to him. But when I explain what's happened, he shakes his head.

'I am *so* sorry,' he says. 'I completely forgot to pack tape this morning.' An error for which I can hardly give him a hard time. I should probably have thought to pack some myself.

I soldier on. As the miles pass the pain subsides a little. Or perhaps just becomes less of a focus of attention because of the pain I'm now experiencing in my shoulders. But I keep my chin up – this is nothing worse than I experienced wheeling around Wellingborough – and when at mile ten I trap my little finger in the wheel again, it concentrates my mind wonderfully. I have to focus so hard on making sure it doesn't happen again that the remainder of the race – even the punishing incline at the end – passes in what's probably a very timely blur.

Seeing the finish line, even though I'm breathing hard, spluttering and coughing, gives me a real boost and I cover the final yards without faltering; but almost the second I cross the line, I roll to a stop, exhausted. And the minute I see my family rushing towards me, I don't mind admitting that I burst into tears.

Matt gets to me first, throwing his arms around me and giving me a bear hug. 'Well done, Dad,' he says. 'You did so well!'

I can barely mumble more than a 'Thanks, Mattie', I'm so overwhelmed. So proud to have achieved what I've achieved, obviously, but even prouder that my boy is there to greet me.

Lisa, Amy and Ellie are right behind him, and now we all hug. I don't think there can be a better feeling for a man in the whole world. Ellie's still got her sign, now much crumpled, and it crumples even more when I gather her up onto my lap.

'Are you tired?' she wants to know as she snakes her arms round my sweaty neck.

'Yes, sweetheart,' I tell her. 'I'm exhausted. But I'm all excited and happy at the same time.'

'Why?' Typical Ellie. Time for the usual 20 questions.

'Why am I tired?'

She shakes her head. 'No, silly Daddy. Why are you excited and happy?'

'Because', I say, 'I have just pushed my wheelchair over 13 miles, and that is a *very* long way!' And it is. I can't take it in, really. The most I have pushed myself, ever, has been 5 miles around Wellingborough, and it's only now I'm done that I really appreciate what a long way I have travelled. I've just done something I really thought I never would – never could – do, and I'm overwhelmed to think that now I have.

'Do you get a medal for that?' Ellie's now asking me, pragmatically.

'Of course he does,' Amy reassures her. 'And a goody bag, as well. I saw them.'

'A goody bag?' says Ellie, down off my lap like an Exocet.

'Yes, with stuff in it,' Amy says, as she leads the procession back to the finish so that we can bag one. 'Maybe sweets.'

That's it, then. A-goody-bag-hunting we must go. 'And Dad's medal, don't forget!' Lisa says.

12 March 2012

Number of miles needed to be wheeled today by Nigel: At a guess, about 0.001.

Number of miles wheelable by Nigel today: Absolutely definitely 0.0000000001.

Though, on the plus side, number of times it will be necessary to pass that frigging jigsaw, as a consequence – oh, joy of joys: 0.

Now I get it. This is where, as they say in the film *Fame*, you start paying. My arms feel as though someone affixed a brace of medicine balls to them in the small hours; my back is protesting so much you could probably hear the creaks in Calais; and my fingers – particularly my pinkies – look like Wall's finest. So far so expected, as every half-marathon veteran knows. And it's both a curse and a source of pride all at once.

But it's my inner thighs that are giving me the most cause for consternation, because I simply can't fathom why they hurt so much. Oh, but how they do! I decide to give myself the day off to sit around wincing, soaking up the plaudits and feeling smug. Heck, I might even see how soon I can register for next year.

13 March 2012

Jigsaw? What jigsaw? CANNOT MOVE.

Scrub that last entry. I am now IN AGONY. Though I have at least worked out why my thighs hurt so much. Why hadn't I realized? It was those water bottles I carried round with me! I've just worked out that I wheeled 13.1 miles yesterday with two of them clamped permanently between my knees. I hear that women pay good money for personal trainers to give them that kind of sustained workout. Am expecting compliments all round on my newly svelte legs. Though that's really no consolation.

'What you need,' Lisa tells me, 'is a massage.' And handily we have a friend, Shirley Marriot, who's a professional sports masseuse. Perhaps as much to do something about my permanent wincing expression as my legs, Lisa calls her up and, bless her, she comes straight over. She then spends the best part of an hour going to work on my arms, back and legs, and though she finds muscles in the latter that I didn't even know I had (and neither did they, evidently, given the amount they are protesting), I feel so much better after she's done with me.

Better enough, in fact, to pop into town and catch up with my friend Darren, at Wellingborough Cycles, who kindly made himself available to be on hand during the half marathon, in case I had any issues with my wheelchair. When I tell him how stiff I've been, he has another solution: a sports supplement.

'Try this,' he says, handing me a bottle that's a quarter full of yellowish powder. 'It's designed to take after you've just done a strenuous event.'

I take his word for it, take it home and mix it up as per the instructions. It's vile. It says on the bottle that it's banana flavoured, but if so, it's like no banana I've ever come across in my life.

I force it down anyway, like the serious athlete I now am.

14 March 2012

I always knew it wouldn't be long before I cracked, and I do. Today I log on to my page on the JustGiving website and find I've already managed to raise over £575 for CMT United Kingdom. I've earned a really big bar of chocolate. I must have burned loads of calories, after all. And what my sports-mad brother doesn't know about my post-marathon diet cannot hurt him …

Looking at the website, and the image of my face grinning out, I find my thoughts drift away, to Mum and Dad. I know there have been all sorts of times along the way when I've missed them, but there's something about having achieved something as gruelling as that half marathon that makes me really wish they could both be here to see it. I do some sums. Dad would have been 83 last month, Mum 81. And whereas she's been gone over three years, he's now been gone three decades. He was 54 when he died – only a few years older than I am now.

I owe such a debt of gratitude to my parents. I owe so much to Lisa, of course – my wife has been and always will be my soulmate and my rock – but also to the parents who gave me the will and enthusiasm to succeed when I was growing up, no matter what challenges I had to face. They were always so supportive, so loving, and had such a brilliant attitude. I can hear them saying it now: 'Nigel, you don't know what you can do until you try.'

And they let me try. From day one, they never stopped me from trying. Hard though it must have been to watch me struggle – particularly for my mum, who must have been permanently on pins, worrying that I'd hurt myself – they let me, in order that I could work out for myself what I could and couldn't do. Sure, there were occasions when I miscalculated and made a fool of myself – who doesn't? – but trying and failing, and then trying a different way, is how, ultimately, you succeed.

'Having a go' was something Dad always encouraged, even when his own dignity was at stake.

He was a competent golfer – he'd taken up golf as a way of de-stressing – and I remember when I was about 16 or 17 going to the golf course with him, so that I could keep him company and see what golf was all about.

So we trundled round with his golf cart, the pair of us. Before long I felt emboldened enough to want to try it for myself.

'Can I have a go?' I asked him, when we were about half-way round the course.

'Sure,' he said, grinning. 'Here you are.'

He handed me a seven iron, and showed me the correct way to stand and hold it. Naturally, this wasn't the easiest thing to do, because of my poor balance, but eventually I got settled and swung the club as he directed, bracing myself excitedly for the hefty slug of metal on golf ball.

Sadly, no such satisfying slug was forthcoming. Instead, the club touched the ball by no more than a gnat's whisker, causing it to plop off the tee and dribble to a stop a few inches in front of me.

The club, however, had by now gathered plenty of momentum and, undeterred by its failure to launch the ball skywards, flew from my hands (which had, probably in disappointment, relaxed their grip on it) up into the air and towards the distant treeline.

To his credit, my dad didn't laugh out loud (or, conversely, stress about his expensive seven iron), but instead followed its trajectory to where it thumped back down onto the fairway. 'You know,' he said, as straight-faced as he could manage under the circumstances, 'that's the furthest I think I've ever seen a club travel.'

My dad died in 1983. And as with all life-changing events, I remember it clearly. It was a sunny day in October, and, having taken early retirement, Dad was out in the garden, as he often was in those days, taking advantage of the unexpectedly balmy weather by doing a bit of pre-winter pruning and tidying up.

I was in the kitchen when he came in and complained to Mum of chest pains, and I watched her calmly get some pills out and slip one into his mouth, under his tongue. I'd find out later that he'd recently been having heart palpitations, but at this point I knew nothing about them. All I knew was that he was sitting there, looking pale, clutching his arm – he was obviously in a lot of pain – while someone, perhaps my mum, perhaps one of my elder brothers, went out into the hall to call an ambulance.

I went into the living room then, feeling useless and anxious, panicking and at a loss to know what I could do to help. There was nothing I *could* do, of course, bar watch the ambulance pull up outside and the paramedics load Dad into it and, as I watched it speed off with both my mother and father, pray that everything was going to be OK.

I never expected my father to die. Why would I, when he was only 54? Anyway, within a few hours of his being admitted the news was encouraging. Mum called home to say he'd had a mild heart attack, and that things were stable, which meant we could go and visit him later on. Which we did, and I was pleased to see him sitting up in bed, looking tired, yes, but very happy to see us all.

When we returned the following day to find him lying down and a little pale, I just thought he was tired from both his ordeal the previous day and the night spent in an uncomfortable hospital bed (I obviously had experience in this regard). I never even really read anything into the way he said goodnight to me. 'Goodbye, Nigel,' he said, in what seemed such a formal voice.

The call from the ward sister came in the middle of the night, the sound of the phone so jangling and insistent in the silence that all of us – jolted awake, imagining Mum scrabbling for her dressing gown – now understood that suddenly this was serious. Phones don't ring in the small hours for any other reason.

I remember watching helplessly as Gary helped Mum into his car and they drove away, my heart thumping in my chest as I stood in the doorway. My sister was in college then, so I was alone in the house, and as I perched on the sofa, close to the telephone, waiting for news, I don't think I can remember ever feeling quite so alone and scared.

I remember desperately trying to find something to occupy my mind, and focusing – almost desperately – on my upcoming 21st birthday and what kind of party I might have. It didn't help a great deal, but at least it was something. I had been excited about my coming of age for a long time, and somehow – even though I knew that rationally it was ridiculous – to focus on it made me feel slightly more hopeful; if I wished it enough, wished hard for my dad to be there, then surely, *surely*, he wouldn't die on me.

I heard the key in the front door an hour or so later. I think I knew then – they had been gone for such a short time – that they had been too late: that my father had left us. Mum was shaking as she walked in, half propped up by Gary. 'Oh, love,' she said, crying. 'Your dad's gone.'

I had never in my life known pain like it. My hero, my supporter, my father, my friend. Gone. Gone forever. The pain was indescribable. Unbearable. I know I only bore it because my brothers were both heroes. They were hurting as much as we all were, but they kept things together. Supported Mum, supported me, supported Nicola, supported all of us; they were

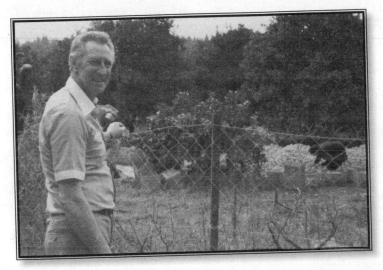

Dad, a year before he passed.

a testament to the strength of the father we'd lost. He would have been so proud of the way they helped me and guided me, even if, being the age I was, and having that over-cockiness of youth, I wasn't always the most receptive of listeners.

He would have been proud of Mum, too, because though she'd lost her husband at such a tragically early age, she managed to pull herself together and carry on courageously. She must have been so lonely – by now I was the only one living at home, and I was mostly out at work – but she retained her independence and refused to mope. And though Dad had always dealt with what in those days were the traditionally male roles – the mortgage, the finances, the insurance and so on – she stepped up to the plate and dealt with everything. When I look back at how my mum coped with having her life changed irrevocably at a time no one would expect, it reminds me how important it is to count blessings daily.

26 March 2012

Fraction of jigsaw now completed: I'd say roughly a good eighth.
Percentage of corners gone missing: An incontrovertible 25.
Percentage of enthusiasm for going through the hoover bag
*   again: Single figure. Low single figure.*

Another challenge involving Ian Blackett today, but this time there's no danger of him sustaining a head injury. We're off to pay a visit to a lady called Etam Dedhar. Etam runs a bespoke cake-making business near where we live. She emailed me to say that she'd heard about The 50 List, and thought she'd get in touch to see if I'd like her to help me achieve one of my challenges. Would that be of interest, she wondered? You bet. So now we're all set: Ian's going to come along and record me learning how to make a decent crème brûlée.

The crème brûlée is – and I'll accept no arguments on this point – the best dessert ever. One of my old work colleagues and I used to go to a great pub called the Spencer Arms in Chapel Brampton in Northampton, and even if we didn't have time to sit down and have a proper lunch, we'd barely ever leave without having one of theirs. Crème brûlée is to die for, every single time.

Like lots of other people, however, I never thought I'd make one myself. For I am not, shall we say, the most able of cooks. If anyone enquires on the subject, I tell them my cooking skills are legendary – all they need to do is ask any fireman.

Actually, I'm not that bad. I can make a mean soufflé omelette (not nearly as difficult as the name suggests) and my prawn and chicken green Thai curry is pretty good as well. I am also conversant with all the trendy ingredients of the moment and can deploy pesto, peppery salad leaves, toasted pine nuts, chilli, lemon and coriander not only with aplomb but also in the same salad all at once. And here's a tip for free (OK, it's from my friend David Kirby): unexpected though it may seem, the humble nectarine goes brilliantly with basil and cherry tomatoes.

But I know and accept my limitations. Give me a one-pan situation or a salad to assemble and I can rise to the challenge every time. But there are two key things that stop me from applying to go on *Masterchef*: one is that I am absolutely hopeless at timings (orchestrating a roast dinner would reduce me to a blubbering wreck) and the second is that with wrists and hands that won't do what they're told, I can't heft pots around like Jamie Oliver.

I have one signature dish, though: a Nigel Holland original called Cinder Lamb. Sadly, I'm never asked to make it, but if you want some pointers, just place a whole leg of lamb in a combi oven – you know, the kind where the dial goes to either 'oven' or 'grill'. Plan on turning it to the former – for a lingering, mouth-watering, tender, slow cook – but (this is key) turn it to the other. Trust me. Works brilliantly every time.

It's no wonder, then, that Lisa does most of the serious cooking in our house, and her ginger chicken (not to mention her roasts and her banana cheesecake) are legends far more likely to endure. And no wonder that it never occurred to me to attempt my own crème brûlée. I always thought it was such a timing-heavy, technical and cheffy business, the sort of cookery that, should you blink at the wrong moment (or attempt to make it on a Tuesday, say, in Doncaster, wearing jodhpurs, carrying a pineapple, having first read *War and Peace*, when there's an R in the month and so on), the whole thing would go pear-shaped at a stroke. Yes, *that* kind of cheffy. So why bother?

But having decided that its very complexity made it a dead cert for The 50 List, I've since learned (though don't tell a soul about this, obviously) that it's apparently not that difficult at all. Not if you have the benefit of some proper guidance, anyway. And a really cracking recipe, of course …

Etam's Amazing Crème Brûlée

4 egg yolks
55g (2oz) sugar
130ml (5fl oz) milk
300ml (10fl oz) cream
1 vanilla pod

1. Preheat the oven to 140°C/275°F/Gas Mark 1.
2. Whisk together the egg yolks and sugar.
3. Heat the milk and cream and add the extracted seeds from the vanilla pod.

4. Put on the heat and bring to a point just before boiling.
5. Pour through a sieve onto the egg and sugar mixture while whisking.
6. Place four to five ramekins on a 3-inch-deep tray lined with a towel (this will stop the ramekins sliding about when you put the tray in the oven).
7. Pour the mixture into the ramekins.
8. Pour boiling water into the tray until the water level comes up two-thirds of the side of the ramekins.
9. Put the tray into the oven, on the middle shelf. After 30 minutes give the tray a little shake to see if the custard mix has set. If it wobbles, it's set.
10. Take out of the oven and let the ramekins sit to cool before putting them in the fridge.
11. When you're ready to serve, sprinkle a layer of caster sugar evenly over the set custard. Using a culinary torch (or mini flame thrower), heat the sugar until it melts. Don't overheat it, as the sugar will burn and taste bitter.

I can't tell you how good my first ever crème brûlée tasted. And when I say I can't, I mean it. Yes, I did plenty of tasting of it – before, during and after – but the finished creations, lovingly transported back into the bosom of my family, were devoured by the kids at a stroke.

Nigella, eat your heart out. Here comes Nigel!

APRIL

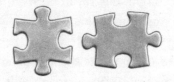

14 April 2012

Quote for the day: 'The best laid plans of mice and men ...'

And how does that other quote go? Ah yes, something about March winds and April showers, if I recall. Which is apt, because it's definitely decided to rain on my parade. I am sitting on a bed in an examination room in hospital and I have a headache. Correction: I *still* have a headache.

I've had a headache on and off now for the best part of a fortnight, which has been annoying, yes, but not particularly worrying. I've still not quite shaken that wretched cold out of my sinuses, so I've naturally been putting it down to that.

I've been bunged up as well. At night particularly. So much so that I've been driving Lisa mad, because I haven't been able to breathe out of either nostril. But today there's been something of a development: one of my eyelids is drooping.

'Can you see that, love?' I asked her when I noticed it. 'Does my left eyelid look droopy to you?'

Lisa inspected it. She is a nurse, so she's good at that. 'Yes, I can,' she agreed. 'How odd. I wonder why that is?'

And, as wives and nurses do, she then inspected me some more. My temple on that side was tender as well, I realized. Had been all morning, come to that.

'And look,' Lisa said, directing my gaze to the bedroom mirror, 'your pupils are unequal as well. Can you see that? The left one is smaller. Have you got any problems with your vision?'

I looked, and saw that she was right. One of my pupils was indeed smaller – the left one, on the same side where my head was so tender and my eyelid was unaccountably droopy. Neither of us had a clue why that might be, so rather than spend hours speculating and performing amateur eye tests, I called NHS Direct.

'Tell me your symptoms,' the lady asked me, but I'd barely even started before she stopped me, having picked up on the 'small pupil' bit immediately.

'A&E,' she said decisively. 'I recommend you get to hospital as a matter of urgency. It might be nothing, obviously, but ...'

She didn't really need to finish the sentence. When someone tells you to get to A&E as a matter of urgency, you don't tend to focus so well on whatever it is they say next. What could possibly be wrong with me? I dreaded to think. So I tried not to, even though my mind was shrieking 'Stroke! Stroke! You might be having a stroke!' at me.

The important thing at this moment, clearly, was not to panic but to get to the place where they could do something more proactive so, leaving Matt and Ellie watching telly, Lisa, Amy and I (Amy was insistent she come with us) jumped into the car to go to hospital.

Here, once again, the words 'small pupil' worked like a charm, and I was whisked – and, yes, that is probably the word for it – up to the high-dependency unit. By now I was no longer scared. I was extremely scared. There are few reasons in life to be allowed to queue jump in a hospital casualty, and they are not generally reasons many would covet. Was I that sick that they thought I might keel over imminently? I tried to make light of it, but the odds seemed to be stacking up against me. Oh, for the reassurance of a solid three-hour wait, clutching one of those tickets you also get in supermarket delis and being grumpy about the vend-ing-machine coffee …

The doctor arrived shortly afterwards. He was a big man with a deep, booming voice and a something-o-scope, with which, having asked me half a dozen probing questions, he examined the pupils of both my eyes.

'CT scan,' he said finally. 'We need to perform a CT scan, so that we can see what's going on in there.'

Once again, this was not the best news I could hear. Though it didn't involve needles it did involve the words 'CT scan', which was reason enough to alarm me even more. I knew Lisa could see that too, despite her constant reassurance that there could be all sorts of reasons that weren't seri-ous in the least, and despite her telling me I must keep calm and not second guess. And I did try to keep calm – primarily for Amy, so her being with us was undoubtedly a good thing.

'There'll be a bit of a wait,' the doctor went on, 'because the CT team aren't in at weekends, so we've had to call in the on-call technician specially.'

At this news, of course, despite my very best intentions, my anxiety reached DEFCON 5. It took a real effort of will to keep my tone light. I'd be fine, I assured Lisa; she and Amy should go home and they should all have something to eat. Matt and Ellie would be hungry, after all, wouldn't they? Yes, definitely better that she come back later on. Funny how you do that; how you strive to maintain normality in such situations. To refuse to accept that something serious might be going on. But it might be, even so.

So here I am. Two hours have passed and, on the plus side, I haven't keeled over. But at the same time the pain in my head isn't any better, and I can't stop my brain from working overtime. I'm normally such a 'glass half full' kind of guy, someone who always looks on the bright side. But as I stack up the symptoms beside the professionals' response to those symptoms, I can't help but dwell on all the worst-case scenarios. What if it's this? What if it's that? What if it's even worse – what if it's the *other*? Despite my trying really hard to think about something else entirely, my mind has other ideas. Words like 'brain haemorrhage', 'tumour' and 'stroke' keep swirling round, like the front runners in some scary beauty parade of every life-threatening illness I've ever heard of. And there's another question: why? Which generates lots of other little sub-questions. Why me? Why now? Why when I'm having so much fun? Why when I'm in the middle of such a big personal challenge? I can't be ill now – I don't have time to be. I can't *die!*

By the time someone returns to take me down for my CT scan I am finding it increasingly hard not to have cast myself in a tragic role in *Casualty*, a television programme I generally don't much enjoy, on account of being married to an ex-nurse who tells you everything before it happens. Oh, how I wish she were here now, even though it was I who told her to go ... I need her to be calm and stoical for both of us.

At least now something is happening. I have something else to focus on – principally a giant white Polo mint, which, once I'm on the platform and my head is strapped in place so that I can't move it, glides across and swallows me up.

The wait afterwards isn't a lengthy one. And there's a sliver of encouraging news.

'We can't see anything noticeable on the scan,' the doctor tells me, reassuringly. 'But then again,' he adds, frowning, 'you might have had a bleed that the scan couldn't pick up. So the next step – because there obviously is *something* going on in there – is to investigate further via a lumbar puncture.'

By now, though, on the outside I'm a nodding and smiling Mr Cool, on the inside my stomach is in knots. I know about lumbar punctures – enough to know this will mean an overnight stay in hospital. I also know they are not procedures that are done lightly. The reassurance of the scan coming back negative begins to evaporate. Just because they didn't find anything doesn't mean it doesn't exist. It clearly does, or else why this new procedure? The question is: what exactly is the 'it'?

It's yet another doctor, once I've been transferred up to a ward, who seems to want to try to pin it down for me. He's really thorough in his visual examination of my eyes, tracking them by having me follow his finger left and right, up and down, round and round, and having done so, he says, 'I know what this is.'

Then he seems to completely contradict himself. I'm so tense that a lot of what he explains washes over me, but at least I pick up the words that matter. It could be related to my CMT, it could be an extreme example of a migraine, but – and just when I'm starting to exhale just a little, too – it could equally be an aneurysm or another kind of brain bleed.

I'm terrified. I don't think I've ever felt so alone. What I want, more than anything, is Lisa to be beside me and – I'm not ashamed to admit it – hold my hand.

There is good news of a sort, however. Because the consultant is so confident he's narrowed down the cause of my symptoms, he goes on to tell me I won't need the lumbar puncture after all. But I will need to stay in hospital over the weekend, even so. This is potentially serious, and it would be insane to go home, clearly. Then, come Monday, assuming there's no escalation in my condition in the meantime, I will have further investigations by an opthalmologist and a neurologist, from which the root of the problem will, the consultant hopes, be fully ascertained.

I call Lisa to tell her and find that she's already on her way, which means she has to return home to get some overnight things for me, which means I have to wait for her a little longer. But when she arrives (a joy in itself; just seeing her 'You'll be fine' look calms me) I see she's even thought to bring my iPad. I'm really grateful that thought occurred to her, as

I'm on a ward that, because of its transient nature, has no bedside radios or TVs.

I am in with a real mix of patients, in what's known as a short-stay ward, which is where you get put while in transit from A&E. From here either you get moved up to the appropriate medical or surgical ward or you get discharged, so we're a pretty disparate bunch.

It's a big ward – five bays in all, with four patients in each. I feel lucky not only that the chap in the bed next to mine is around my own age but also that we seem to have a great deal in common. We talk for most of the evening – non-stop, pretty much, about a shared passion for Formula 1 and motorsport generally. He also shares my enthusiasm for drag racing and fast road cars, and his company is a real pick-me-up. By the time it's 'lights out', I find that despite regular blood pressure, blood oxygen and temperature checks, I've not thought about what might be wrong with me for ages.

Naturally, this being a hospital, I don't sleep well. I'm uncomfortable, hot and, with two heart patients in the bay, driven half mad by the constant beep of heart monitors. Almost as soon as I drift off, the relative silence (the monitors have eventually become white noise) is broken again at 1.00 a.m. by a young guy being wheeled up from A&E.

By 4.30 a.m. I can't lie there in the bed any longer, and decide to haul myself up into my wheelchair and give up on sleep; I'll do some work instead, I think, on my iPad. I wheel myself out into the corridor near the yellowy glow of the nurses' station, and they don't seem to mind. In fact, they even give me a cup of tea. I spend two hours there, quietly working on my iPad in the pool of light, and one of the nurses explains that the lad who was brought in at 1.00 a.m. was in because of a suicide attempt. It's a sobering thought, and in the small hours, the vulnerable hours, I can't help thinking about him.

15 April 2012

Sunday is supposed to be a day of rest, isn't it? Fat chance of that for the staff, even if the patients are all dozing. In here it's clearly business as usual. I have to hand it to them: the staff are all fantastic. They seem to spend every single moment being rushed off their feet, but at no point do I hear anyone grumbling or complaining – quite the opposite, in fact. They seem always to be on hand, offering help even before it's asked for, and I marvel at how they never seem to get frustrated at the phenomenal amount of work they have to do. The word 'professional' really does seem to still apply in this organization. In fact that feels like an understatement.

But later in the day there's sadness, and again, it really gets to me. The young guy who was brought in last night is now awake, and as I sit listening to his story – one of despair – I feel so sorry for what life has thrown at him. He's so young, and I believe has so much to live for, but he's at rock bottom, so he's blind to the possibilities.

Even more shocking is what I hear from the guy I got to know yesterday. He's quite candid. He tells me he's also in hospital as a result of a failed suicide bid. He lives alone and in a very matter-of-fact manner tells me that once he gets home he'll probably not want to come out again.

I feel helpless and don't really know what to say. What *can* you say that won't come out as a platitude? I wish him well. I really hope he gets better.

In the afternoon I'm seen again by the consultant. After examining me again and seeming not at all concerned by the end, he tells me he's going to arrange for me to have an MRI scan on Monday, so that they can take a proper look at my carotid artery. They want to ascertain if it's been damaged in such a way as to cause a blood clot to break free and enter my brain. They are also going to X-ray my chest to see if the nerves look OK, but as there seems no urgency to any of this I feel immeasurably reassured; had they felt the need to do it now, they would have made it happen.

All of which leaves me free to eat – no procedures, no nil by mouth – and watch several movies back to back (all hail that mighty iPad). I have roast chicken with all the trimmings followed by two desserts: a fruit jelly (which I know Ellie would love) and a delicious-looking caramel mousse that wouldn't look out of place in a fancy restaurant. If it weren't for the constant blood-pressure checks and the reality check of hearing about my fellow patients, it could be a relaxing stay in a hotel.

But not that relaxing. Though my headache's eased now that I've been given some stronger painkillers, the undercurrent of anxiety persists. When Lisa and the children arrive I greet them as if they are long-lost relatives just returned from an expedition to the Galapagos. Such a short time apart but how long it's felt!

I can see Lisa's worried, but she goes straight into professional mode, radiating calm and explaining the medical terminology. The kids look calm, too – their mother's influence, I'm sure. And, naturally, Ellie gets the jelly.

16 April 2012

I must be acclimatizing now because when I wake on Monday morning, I have at least had a couple of hours of unbroken sleep. And I'm still here – no sudden seizure, no collapse, no other crisis – and though I still have my headache I no longer have the constant gnawing butterflies every time I wonder what might be wrong with me.

'Good morning, Nigel!' the healthcare assistant with the tea trolley says to me. 'How are you today? Would you like a cup of tea?'

It's the same when another lady rolls along, bearing breakfast. 'Morning, Nigel!' she says, in the same cheerful voice. 'Which would you prefer – cereal or toast?'

I love the way they do that – make the effort to call you by your name. It's not that difficult to find out; it's up there above your bed, after all. The fact that they bother makes all the difference.

My chest X-ray is done mid-morning. It takes very little time and, since I've still not keeled over, I'm beginning to feel cautiously confident that, once the MRI is done, there's a good chance I'll be able to go home. After all, though the pupil size hasn't increased, it's not worsened. Which surely means something.

There is one small ordeal I have overlooked regarding the MRI, however. As the nurse patiently explains, to my growing dismay, someone is soon going to come and put a needle in my arm.

'It's a cannula,' she explains. 'You need it there so that they can put the dye in.' This is the dye that they are going to inject into my body so that the MRI can see the web of arteries clearly. This naturally sends me into a quiet, unassuming but nevertheless complete meltdown. I've been eating lunch, but my appetite is no more.

She goes then, but immediately I call her back. I have to.

'I have a phobia of needles,' I explain. 'I'm really sorry, but –'

'Oh, you poor thing,' she says, immediately making me feel 100 per cent better. 'Would you like me to do it for you instead?'

I'm so grateful. It might be nothing much to most people, but just the fact that she's taken my blood pressure several times and is a friendly, familiar face helps a lot.

She does a great job, being sensitive to a problem she probably comes across often, letting me know when it's going in but making sure I don't actually see it, and before I know it the thing is in and I'm off down to the MRI scanner, where I have to transfer to a special-issue non-magnetic wheelchair, to avoid the possibility of both it and me flying though the air, Superman-style. As it happens, my chair's titanium, so it's one of the few that aren't magnetic, but I can't vouch for the odd nut or bolt here and there, and pushing my luck isn't on today's agenda.

It's a complicated business being prepared to go into an MRI scanner. I'm put on a gurney, which will slide me head first into the tunnel, which from my new position I now see looks very small.

'It *is* small,' warns the technician, 'and the only thing you'll be able to see once you're in there is the tunnel wall, just above your face. So I'm going to fix an angled mirror up so that you don't get too claustrophobic; it'll let you see out better, into the room.'

He puts a contraption over my face that contains the promised mirror, and now I can see feet and the door. I wasn't feeling claustrophobic till he mentioned the word 'claustrophobic'. Now I am a bit. I think I'll probably just close my eyes.

'Right,' he says cheerily. 'Now I have to fit a long tube to your cannula.' Ah, the cannula. 'Which will be connected to the pump, which will inject into you the special fluid that will be picked up by the scanner. OK?'

'OK,' I say, my voice muffled by the mirror contraption.

'Now the headphones.' He slips a pair carefully over my ears. 'Choice of music?'

'Choice of music?' This is a new one on me.

'Yes, we always play you music. It's to drown out the noise. It's the magnets. They are *very* noisy. It'll help muffle them a bit.'

Oh, I see. 'Erm, what have you got?' I ask him. 'I can cope with anything as long as it's not Barry Manilow.'

'What's your favourite?'

'Have you got some Kaiser Chiefs?'

'You know what? I think we do.'

So that's me set, I think, as I start my slow horizontal journey into the scanning tunnel. Eyes tight shut. Earphones on. Humming along to 'I Predict a Riot'. I can cope with this, I'm sure. Then I wait. And I wait. And I wait a little more. Then I remember him telling me that it's OK to talk to them, as they can hear me.

'Er, has it started yet?' I ask. No answer.

I wait some more. 'Er, hello, has it started yet?'

Again nothing. Then a thought pops into my brain. I didn't actually see him attaching the tube to my cannula. Only felt it. What if the tube has nothing in it but air? It's the sort of irrational thought that assaults you when you least expect it, and it makes me feel suddenly panicky. What if they pump air into my arm? Won't I die?

'Hello?' I say. Actually, to be honest, it's more of a squeak.

Still nothing. So I decide to flap my legs around instead. I'm not *exactly* panicking. Just becoming a little agitated. OK, a lot agitated. In any event, it has two of them rushing in to see if I'm OK. Seems they just forgot to turn the sound up or something. Panic over. Well, that's the impression I'm keen to give them, anyway.

The scan itself is over quicker than I expect. Yes, it is *incredibly* noisy, but being a speed freak I'm used to those kinds of decibels, and it seems I've barely got into full humming flow before the noise stops and the gurney rolls back out again.

That was actually OK, I think, as I'm wheeled back onto the ward to await the results with Lisa. I don't know if it's just the reassurance of having her with me, but by now I feel surer and surer that they're not going to be the horror of my earlier imaginings.

But perhaps I am wrong.

'Hello,' says a woman who seems to have appeared out of nowhere. She is in her forties, I'd say, and wearing a white uniform. Like a nurse, but very slightly different. In her hand, I also notice, she carries a bunch of leaflets, one of which she now thrusts in my direction.

'You must be Nigel. I'm from the Stroke Services team,' she says.

I almost choke. STROKE? Did I hear her right? *Stroke?* I'm immediately overcome by a feeling of cold dread. What does she know that I don't? Have they given her the results before me? Have I had – am I going to have – a *stroke?*

I'm so lost for words that perhaps she thinks I've already lost the power of speech. Whatever. She smiles at Lisa and me and glides on.

'Of course she doesn't know anything you don't,' Lisa chides me. 'Don't be silly. She's just doing the rounds. This is a ward full of stroke patients, so it's an easy mistake to make.' She nods towards my wheelchair. 'See?'

I feel a bit better. A bit, I'll concede. But not a lot.

Not much at all, as it turns out, because I can't help thinking the worst, with or without the wretched pamphlet. By the time the doctor arrives, I am visibly shaking. Almost nauseous, I am so scared by this point. Not so much by my current condition

(I don't feel half as bad as I did on Saturday) but by the implications, the potential, the ticking bomb inside my head.

'Nothing wrong,' says the doctor cheerily. 'Can't see a thing.' He pulls the curtains and perches on the corner of the bed. 'We think it's probably Horner's syndrome, all things considered.'

'So not a stroke?'

He smiles. 'No, not a stroke.'

He goes on to explain what Horner's syndrome is: in essence a condition that can be brought on by a number of different factors, but which typically, when investigated, throws up negative results. The 'can't see a thing' situation. It might be, he suggests, that there's been a dissection of my carotid artery, causing the symptoms, but that the artery itself has now healed.

And he seems perfectly calm, and not at all worried. Fingers crossed it stays that way ...

17 April 2012

To my great relief, it does stay that way. Better than that, even: although my pupil isn't yet back to normal, my headache has now completely gone, as has the tenderness at the side of my face. Which must be a positive, surely?

'Yes,' says the consultant when he comes to see me today. Better still, he pronounces me good to go.

'We'll see you in three months,' he says. 'Sooner, of course, should any of your problems reappear. But, yes, you're good to go.'

'See,' Lisa says, as we drive home at lunchtime. 'I told you everything would be OK.'

'Did you always think that?' I ask her. 'I mean, *really*?'

She smiles. 'A lot of people have been praying for you at church, Nigel.'

I'm not sure what to say to that. Not even sure what to think. Does praying make a difference? I wish I knew.

Or, actually, when I think about it, perhaps it's best that I don't know. All I know is that I'm very, very thankful.

*   *   *

I suppose God, religion, the idea of heaven and hell, and all the rest of it, were not concepts that troubled me much, growing up. I was raised, as most people in Britain were in the 1960s, in a loosely but reassuringly traditional Christian fashion. Christian in the sense that we were Church of England, at any rate. My mum and dad really weren't churchgoers. Bar Mum's attendance at the odd Christmas Eve service, weddings and funerals were pretty much the extent of it. But my schooling was firmly traditional and of its time. We had assembly every morning, said grace before lunch, had harvest festival and sang carols at Christmas – though, as already recorded, my star turn in the school nativity play had little to do with the birth of baby Jesus.

By my teens I was beginning to enjoy more earthly pleasures, and at the age of 16 – a little younger than many of my contemporaries – I began to really spread my wings a bit.

It was at that age that I left Martindale School and transferred to a residential college geared to those with disabilities:

Hereward College, in Coventry. I had always wanted to study chemistry, physics and biology, but my grades weren't quite good enough for it to be clear I'd succeed at them, so I was advised to stick with what I was good at: business and commerce.

And they were right, in that I did get good grades in those subjects, but a part of me will always wonder what I might have done, career-wise, had I put my foot down and insisted. Either become a scientist or blown up a lab, I suppose. If I'm honest, I suppose probably the latter.

Once again, a big focus at college was sport. I took up swimming pretty seriously, I competed once again at Stoke Mandeville, and I also joined the table tennis team. At this time of my life my disability was pretty stable, and I remember thinking often how lucky I'd turned out to be in the scheme of things; compared to some of my friends at Martindale I had got off so lightly. I was shocked to hear, after only a few months up in Coventry, that no fewer than three of my good friends had passed away

In contrast I was loving my first taste of real independence. While my old mates from home were still living with their parents, I had the sort of freedom most wouldn't see till they were older – the sort of freedom kids first taste when going to university today. As we all lived together, on site, in big blocks of student halls, socializing and making friends was easy. We were well served in that respect, as the halls were well equipped; we had a television room, a pool room and a payphone room (for calling home), as well as a 'quiet' room, which was never very quiet.

I made some good friends pretty quickly, so homesickness wasn't an issue. Neither was money, because we had a once-a-week supplementary allowance paid to us, so, courtesy of social services, we all had £7.50 a week to spend in our favourite haunt, the Woodlands pub across the road.

Looking back, they seem such innocent times, really. Seventeen-year-olds, in a pub, sipping their illicit pints of lager, eating cockles slathered in vinegar and pepper, putting the world to rights all evening ... Well, till the 9.00 p.m. college curfew, that was: if you wanted to stay out till 10.00 p.m. you had to get a special pass. But we didn't bother – we were squiffy on one pint anyway.

While I was at college I also learned to drive – a friend of Dad's taught me – so by the time I had left and began work for Rank Xerox in 1982, I felt I was properly independent, even if I did still have to walk wearing the hated metal calipers, clunking through the office and occasionally squeaking as I passed, and having to oil them with the secretaries' typewriter oil.

This too, however, finally changed for me, and for the better, when, in late 1983, just before my dad passed away, I had my first pair of plastic splints made. Technology had moved on in this area, as in all things, and the splints did exactly the same job as the big, metal calipers, but were, in contrast, incredibly discreet. Finally I could go around without anyone knowing I had an orthotic appliance on each leg. Best of all, though, was that for the first time since I was little more than a toddler, I could wear normal shoes, purchased from a shoe shop. This was an incredible first, though, ironically, I didn't go out and buy new shoes straight away. My dad was a really snappy dresser and I always thought he looked cool, so, as we had the same size feet, I borrowed some of his. It was a nice way to remember my dad, having something of his on my feet, and it still makes me smile to think that the first pair of non-orthotic shoes I ever wore came from his wardrobe. It felt fitting, somehow.

But for all that I was too busy with life on earth to think about God, it seemed he was just biding his time till he could come and find me. If the loss of my dad had hit me brutally and painfully, the years that followed took their toll slowly but just as surely.

I was marking time, really. By the late 1980s, I was working for Middlesex Training Centre, teaching 16–18-year-olds computer studies and basic electronics. This was at the height of the YTS years – the years of the youth training scheme that was so much in vogue at the time, the purpose of which was to try to get unemployed youngsters up to scratch for the workplace. It was a political hot potato; some thought the scheme brilliant, others felt it was cheap labour. The deal was that these youngsters would only get their dole money if they attended.

There were three types of youngsters who attended the training centre: those who had intelligence and enthusiasm; those who had intelligence but no enthusiasm; and those who were slightly lacking in the intelligence department but had enthusiasm by the shedload. And they were all very different to teach. The first group were great, because they soaked up everything I taught them, attended always, and saw the benefit in doing so. The second group, in contrast, were something of a nightmare, because they were the ones who caused trouble; they were intelligent enough to know they had to turn up every day, but, despite that, they could see no benefit in the actual learning bit, so put in no effort, no matter how hard I tried to engage them. The third group were probably the most rewarding. They wanted to learn. They worked hard to grasp the concepts. And when they did understand the subject matter, it was really satisfying to see their growing self-esteem. It was the third group that made it all worthwhile.

Sadly, the reality of my experience with the YTS scheme was that the majority of youngsters who attended were in that second group, which was why, ultimately, my job often got me down.

In some ways I wasn't doing much socially, either. I was a musician, so my life revolved around music. I was either practising my drumming or going to see other bands. You could learn a lot from watching how other drummers played.

Our own band, This Temple Eden, had reached its natural end-point. With the members all off doing new stuff with their lives, musically I was at a bit of a loose end. I still loved playing, and I joined another band, who covered rock songs; but though we rehearsed often, we never actually gigged. It was around that time that Phil Barker, the amazing bassist in my old band, asked me if I'd come along and play drums on a Sunday evening with him at his local church.

It was something I was not at all sure about. So I went along mostly out of curiosity and pragmatism; I would forget the 'church' bit and just see it as another gig. After all, we had a name – we were called Pigs in the Parlour, after a book Phil had read, which I thought was terrifically cool. And I was pleasantly surprised. The songs weren't 'churchy' at all (whatever that meant). They were up tempo and modern, and some even had a rock or jazz funk beat. When I thought about it, I didn't doubt this was down to Phil's influence. He was and is the best bass player I have ever played with or heard. Why wouldn't anything he was involved with be good musically?

Not that I lingered for the middle bit. I loved to play, yes, but they could keep most of the rest of it. I would leave when the preacher – Phil's dad, hence the unlikely connection – stood up and did his preacher bit. Who needed a sermon, after all, when there was a perfectly good pub across the road where I could escape to and have a pint instead?

It was the rain – part of the grand plan? – that held me there one Sunday. The alternative, given that it was pouring down so biblically, would have been to get drenched to the bone. Sitting there, with nothing else to occupy me, I listened, and something weird happened: the words seemed to speak to me.

The spell broken, as it were, I began staying in church for the sermon, and with every Sunday that passed, though I didn't always understand all of it, I found I was beginning to enjoy myself. This was no epiphany – I'm too down to earth, too reluctant to be persuaded by emotions – but I was really beginning to feel that I belonged there.

The timing was obviously perfect. I'd lost my dad just four years earlier and still grieved for him daily, and though my mum was coping – something she always did, with dignity and strength – I knew she missed him dreadfully as well. And she had me to deal with – and by this time I was probably at my most moody. Since Dad had died I'd become steadily disillusioned with life. I really hated my job, which now bored me half to death, and had a wholly negative, stressed outlook. I also, I know, took her terribly for granted at that time and treated home like the proverbial hotel.

So, yes, on reflection, the timing was spot on. I'd just finished playing one day and was preparing to leave when one of my new friends from church said, 'Why don't you invite God into your life?'

To which there was really no answer except: 'What have I got to lose?' It probably wouldn't help (or so my thinking went), but it couldn't do any harm.

My friend gave me a prayer that evening, printed on a plain piece of card, and suggested that I just – well – stand and pray it. So I did. Not then and there – that would have been too excruciating. I knew I'd feel a complete prat reading what he'd given me out loud, and it wasn't rocket science to know that I'd feel a whole lot better if I felt like a prat in the privacy of my own home.

Once I was home, as was the norm on a Sunday night, I felt miserable, knowing that the hated job was all I had to look forward to on Monday. So out came the card and I read what was on it: a short four-line prayer that did what it said on the tin and asked God to come into my life. I read it twice, and both times I had very mixed feelings. Was I standing there talking bollocks or was I about to change my life?

I guessed I'd have to find out in the morning.

18 April 2012

Jigsaw watch: FOUND THE MISSING CORNER! Yes, hot
news just in is that it was under the settee all along
– though, curiously, it was nestling alongside two other
puzzle pieces, neither of which has anything to do with
famous historical steam engines. Hmm. Do my nostrils
catch the faint whiff of espionage?
Indeed not. They catch the whiff of homemade soup ...

I have to convalesce, obviously. That's not up for discussion.
But while I'm banned from doing proper work (as in going to
my office and 'doing some business'), I can at least make some
progress with my list. No, not the newly four-cornered jigsaw,
however much G J Churchward (yes, also a train engineer)
calls to me from the coffee table, but as there is a chicken
carcass going begging in the kitchen today, I decide that I will
come over all cheffy this morning – as befits my new status
– and have a stab at another foodie item on my 50 List: 'Learn
to make proper soup.'

Like many a man who's not a chef by profession, I
have never in my life made a pan of soup. Which is strange,
because soup's such a staple, and such a strong memory
from my childhood. My mum was a superb cook, and
her having homemade soup on the go was a given in our
house. I remember coming in from watching Gary play
football, fingers numb from the cold, nose red and streaming,
and that delicious moment when I'd get that first 'hit' of
aroma.

Is there anything better than dipping chunks of crusty bread into homemade soup? Is there a ready-made soup that could ever compare? Not in my experience.

So it's high time I learned.

Though Lisa is sceptical. 'Without a recipe?' she asks.

'I don't need a recipe,' I tell her. 'I am going to be creative.'

'And what do you plan to create?'

'Chicken and vegetable soup, obviously. We have chicken and we have vegetables. How hard can it be?'

I'm not sure Lisa shares my confidence that I will create a soupy masterpiece, which makes me even more determined to produce exactly that before the children reappear from their various social whirls.

And I have got a recipe in mind, as it happens. I remember seeing it on some cookery show or other – Rick Stein or James Martin, probably, as those two are my favourites – but right now I can only remember a bit of it. I know I could grab one of Lisa's recipe books and follow a recipe line by line, but I've got the bit between my teeth now – that's not learning, that's copying! No, I decide, as Lisa heads off for a well-earned rest with the TV remote, I'm going to fly solo on the soup front. Besides, Delia or Jamie or those two Hairy Bikers would only list a load of ingredients I don't have.

By the time Lisa returns the whole kitchen is wreathed in the sort of rich, wholesome aroma that I imagine you'd aim for if you were selling your house and wanted to create a kind of *Waltons* effect. For I have been busy. I stripped down the chicken carcass, boiled it up and let it simmer, and once it reached the desired level of whatever it was that made it look right (this is all done by professional instinct, of course), I strained it, picked the meat off the bones, sweated leeks and onions in a knob of butter (it's all about sweating – I remember that bit. You definitely mustn't let them colour), and then added the chicken stock, chicken pieces, chopped potatoes, carrots and seasoning, and left it to do what it needed to do. While it was doing that I even managed to find that pesky jigsaw corner piece, which is why soup is the puzzler's best friend.

'That smells gorgeous,' Lisa's forced to admit as she enters the kitchen. I can see she's looking around suspiciously as she speaks.

'You won't find it,' I tell her, as she dips a spoon into the pan and tastes my finished masterpiece. By now I've liquidized it too, leaving just the right amount of lumps.

She licks the spoon and goes, 'Hmmm.' Then looks around again. 'Find what?'

'A cook book,' I tell her. 'This is entirely my own creation.'

She shakes her head. 'I wasn't looking for a cook book,' she says.

'So', I say, perplexed now, 'what are you looking for, then, love?'

She grins. 'What do you think? The stash of empty cans!'

My wife has such a lot of faith in me, doesn't she?

*   *   *

And doesn't faith work in mysterious ways? There was no blinding light, no sudden vision, no shadowy apparition wafting in from the open window. It was just that, for whatever reason – and I was groping for reasons – the week after I'd taken that card home from church, I felt better.

No, work hadn't improved; it was still the same job as ever. It was just that my response to it had changed. And feeling better about that seemed to lead naturally into feeling better about myself, and feeling better about myself made me a much nicer person to be around, which made everything that much better – particularly for my poor, put-upon mum.

The change in how I viewed the world began to reap other rewards. There was no doubt that low morale had crept into the organization for which I was working, but I was soon coping with work so much better. I was feeling positive about it even, and definitely more positive about my students – so much so that in 1988 we even entered several of them into the YTS Training Team of the Year competition. Their task was to impress the judges with their communication and entrepre-neurial skills and, in doing so, demonstrate how good they were at working as a team. I was thrilled when we breezed though the first two rounds of the competition, but I could see that in the final they would be up against some very slick presentations.

But I kept the faith; though our boys weren't perhaps as slick as some of the others to look at (no fancy patter or smart suits and ties), they were very smart – certainly smart enough to win it. And when our name was called out, I couldn't have been more proud.

It was a brilliant prize, which my fellow trainer and I were invited to share with them: a trip to Valencia, in Spain, to visit the Ford factory there, and tickets to the Spanish Grand Prix, as the Ford Motor Company's guests.

But there was an even greater prize waiting for me soon afterwards. One that, ironically, would come about as the result of another fall.

It was in 1990, and I'd gone down one day in the office, hard, and, as was becoming the norm now, required a visit to A&E.

So far, so predictable: a short wait, then a chat with the doctor, followed by an X-ray, then back to wait for the results. But on this day I was particularly lucky. Lucky both in that there wasn't a fracture and in that, surprisingly, the doctor had come across CMT on a few previous occasions and had a good grasp of what the remedy was for soft-tissue injuries. I was accordingly sent off to the physiotherapy department, where I was seen by a young lady called Marianne Webb.

Marianne took a look at my foot and started asking the usual questions. How did I fall? Where did it hurt? Did I do this sort of thing often? As we got chatting, I mentioned that I attended a local church. She told me that her father was a lay reader at another church in Ealing, and suggested that sometime, once my ankle and foot had healed, I might find the time to pop along.

Might I? I weighed up the pros and cons. She was easy going, friendly, approachable and warm. Oh, and she was also the best-looking physiotherapist in the whole place, with a cascade of beautiful dark brown hair. (Though obviously this didn't figure in my thinking at all.) On the other hand, the church was 8.5 miles away.

It was a difficult decision. Took me a full three and a half seconds. On balance, I was pretty certain that I *would* find the time, and once I was properly mobile again – well, my then version of it, anyway – I headed off to St Paul's Church in Northfields, Ealing.

Right away I made an idiot of myself. It was a big old church with what looked like entrances on all sides – there were at least three doors, none of them looking grander than any other, and, as I swiftly found out once I'd parked the car and locked it, none had a sign saying 'entrance'.

I took an educated guess that the entrance would be the door at the front of the building, which looked slightly more imposing than the other two. But for all my tugging and rattling – perhaps it was just stuck – the door refused to allow me inside the church. That was that, then. I had no choice but to go and explore the others, the second of which (and the least prepossessing, in my book) immediately swung open as I pushed it.

I could see my mistake straight away. As could the congregation. I crept inside, blushing hotly under a blaze of dirty looks, for having been the one rattling the back door down in the middle of prayers.

Marianne forgave me, thankfully, and we soon started dating. But, as is the way of things, though I got to know her and her family very well, we were clearly not destined to be together. We're still friends, and good ones – we are godparents to each other's children – and the thing I must thank her for most is for introducing me (once we'd split up, but I was still attending St Paul's) to her old schoolfriend, whose name was Lisa Boyes.

Lisa and I hit it off immediately. She already knew about my CMT, being Marianne's best friend, and right away I could see that she was not the sort of girl to be put off by something as 'superficial' as a disability; she was the sort who was much more interested in the person underneath. Oh, and there was the small matter of my charm and wit, obviously …

Lisa was musical, too, so we had something in common. She was in the church choir – she had a beautiful voice – and had been going to St Paul's since she was at school. She was a student nurse, and in no time at all I was nursing too: nursing an ambition to start going out with her. I loved everything about her. I loved her gorgeous smile, her curly hair, her wonderful laugh, her amazing personality – but most of all I loved the way she'd send me notes (and yes, OK, I'd started it) about just how very much she loved me. She was training in Hammersmith and I would drive over (which was another hike, but I didn't care) at just about every opportunity I could get

Unsurprisingly, given our mutual enthusiasm, we very quickly became an item, and within weeks, as is also the way when you're young and in love, it felt as if we had known each other forever. Though I was soon to be reminded that that wasn't quite the case.

We'd been out to see a band one night (I even recall the band name: Fat and Frantic) and, as we often did, we went back to Lisa's afterwards. We were both starving and I'd suggested that if there were the ingredients in the fridge, I could rustle up some bacon and eggs for us both.

When we arrived and popped our heads round the living-room door, we were greeted by a pretty full house. Lisa's mum had most of the old ladies from her road in for a natter, including Lisa's eccentric 'Auntie Lou' – in reality her great-aunt and sadly in the early stages of Alzheimer's, though we didn't know that then.

'Hello, dear,' Auntie Lou said, as Lisa's mum introduced us.

'Hello,' I said firmly, raising my voice a little. I had already figured out that Auntie Lou must be a little deaf from the way Lisa's mum raised hers when speaking to her. 'Nice to meet you. How are you?'

'Very well,' she said. Then, having finished inspecting me, she smiled and turned back to the group. Which was fine by me, because making small talk with a posse of permed pensioners was no match for a plate of eggs and bacon. Lisa and I backed out of the room again and headed to the kitchen, whereupon, the coast clear, the ladies returned to their chatting, delivering their various verdicts. At least, that's what I imagine must have happened – I couldn't hear exactly what they were saying, obviously. But what I did catch, Lisa's mum having the sort of voice that carries, was, 'Well, he's much better than the last one, for sure!'

So that was that. With the official Boyes seal of approval, I knew I was in this for the long haul. And, in 1992, by which time we'd been together for a couple of years, I decided I would ask Lisa to marry me.

Naturally, because I'm a romantic at heart, I planned my proposal with precision. It was summertime and we were away camping that week, down in Chideock in Dorset, with the Boys' Brigade. Lisa was a staff sergeant – there to help run the camp – and I was one of the 'other halves' who had come to help out where needed, though my official capacity was as drummer for Martin Webb, Marianne's brother, who was also involved in the Boys' Brigade and resident bugler.

It was all very decent and above board; no tent hopping. In fact, I spent the week sharing a tent with one of the senior Boys' Brigade officers, who insisted that of the two tent flaps, only the left-hand one was to be used, as the right-hand one was reserved for emergencies. I'm not sure if this was designed to keep me in at night – using the left one would have meant climbing over him – or just an idiosyncratic preference. Either way, I completely disregarded it, and used whichever flap was nearest. Though not for getting up to any mischief, I hasten to add …

I'd brought my drums down with me, obviously, for the various musical sessions, and my plan for the day (as with all the days we camped there) was to begin early with Martin, jazzing up his reveille with a bit of a drum solo; then, once the day's various activities were over, to walk down to the beach with Lisa that evening, just the two of us, and as the sun set ask her to marry me.

So far, so romantic, but it wasn't quite to be. I got up, as ever, in good time for reveille, crawled out of my tent and headed over to the cookhouse. This being a field, the ground was fairly rutted and uneven, and naturally, my balance having been an issue all my life, traversing it could be something of a challenge. And on this day – as a result of what I think in official circles is called sod's law – it proved too much of a challenge: I fell and hit the deck.

In a re-run of the events that had led me (via Marianne) to Lisa in the first place (an irony that wasn't lost on me), I was spirited off to Bridport Hospital by one of the leaders, Robin Harrison. And in another re-run of that time, I once again got lucky: no bones broken, just the familiar soft-tissue injury.

As I hobbled back into camp, on my standard-issue NHS crutches, it occurred to me that there was now as much chance of me proposing on the beach as there was of Nellie the Elephant taking flight over the Devon coastline. Even if there had been a chance, it was now also raining. And not just raining in a 'cooling the summer heat with a welcome sprinkling of fragrant water' kind of way: it was properly hammering it down, in stair rods, as only an August sky can do. And showing no signs of stopping, either, which you'll know, if you camp on a regular basis, is just about the very last thing to be wished for.

'Shall we go and sit in my car?' I suggested to Lisa once she'd come to find me, which, though perhaps not the most romantic offer she'd ever received, was possibly – no, definitely – the most practical. With the tents all running with water and sagging threateningly in the middle, it was the only place in the whole camp that was warm and dry. Not to mention safe.

'Good idea,' she agreed (she's a girl who knows a decent offer when she sees one), so we headed off and climbed into the car.

Once we were in, I weighed my chances of making the romantic seaside proposal of my imagining and, realizing I had none until my injury was better, I decided to propose to her then and there.

'Lisa?' I said formally, twisting in my seat and adopting what I hoped was a suitably formal tone.

She waited for what was coming, her expression mildly enquiring.

I cleared my throat. I hadn't thought past asking the question and, now that I was about to, it occurred to me that she might say no. I pushed the thought away again. 'I wanted to take you to the beach today and ask you something very important,' I went on. 'But as it is …' I gestured to the rain that was sliding in a solid sheet down the windscreen, 'I have decided to ask you now. Will you marry me?'

There was a heartbeat of a pause, while she digested my little speech. She clearly hadn't had a clue what had been coming. Then she flung her arms around me and almost squeezed the breath from my lungs.

Which I took as a yes. I don't think I've ever felt so happy.

I did things properly. As soon as we returned from our camping trip in Devon, I did what these days some might think old-fashioned, but which I thought was important. I called Lisa's father and asked him for his blessing. I like traditions, and I also thought it was something he would appreciate. He was in his mid-seventies by then, retired from a lifetime as a professional chauffeur, and was very old school. Though by the time I knew him he was an elderly gentleman, who drove everywhere at 30 mph, including motorways, he'd seen active service in the Second World War and had spent time as a prisoner of war both in Italy and in Germany, before being force-marched to freedom by the Russians. I had enormous respect for him. And I'd been right: it really did mean the world to him.

With Bob's blessing secured, we got on with the business of planning our wedding, and Lisa and I were married in St Paul's Church in the spring of 1994.

I was determined to walk my wife back down the aisle without falling over, though with my balance being so poor by then, I knew that unless I had something to lean on, my knees would give way at the drop of a hat. So my good friend Graham Hancock, who managed an aero-modelling shop,

Lisa with her dad.

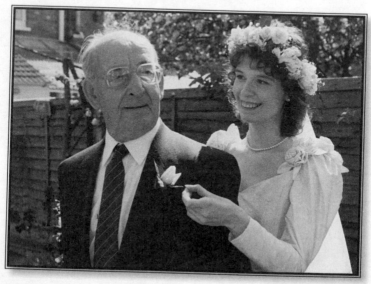

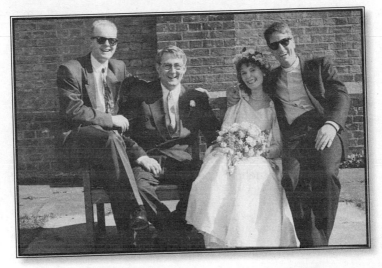

Revd Mike Stewart, me, Lisa and Revd Mark Melluish.
You can never have enough clergy!

took an old walking stick and sawed and hacked away at it for an hour or so, so that my hand – my grip was also now becoming increasingly problematic – could hold it well enough so that I could confidently hold my weight.

I also managed to take Lisa for a spin on the dance floor, as is traditional for newlyweds. Well, I say spin; it was more 'leaning on her and shuffling round in circles'. But I didn't care. I felt immensely proud. Of my wonderful wife, obviously; of myself, for having snared her, but most of all proud to be able to tell the whole world that I was a man who'd dived into marriage with both feet.

And managed not to take a dive in the process.

20 April 2012

Number of activities now completed: 8, and a quarter of a
   jigsaw (and yes, that quarter matters).
Number of boots made for walking: None required, obviously.
But number of wheels made for rolling: A very handy 4.

In the paper once again! I could get used to this, I really could.
This time it's a mention in the *Evening Telegraph*, alerting the
world at large to the fact that, as a part of completing my 50
List, I'm going to take part in the Waendel Walk.

The Waendel Walk is an annual event in Wellingborough,
now in its 34th year. When it began in 1979, it was a one-day
event, offering a choice of two routes around the local environs
– one of a fairly strenuous 29 kilometres and one of a whopping 43. Waendel, by the way, was a person – a Saxon warlord
– and if you want to be a purist, it's actually spelt 'Wændel'. But
these days, like the spelling, the whole thing has stretched out
a bit, and it's a three-day event – or, rather, a series of events,
including cycling and swimming as well as two walks, which
are an altogether more manageable 5 and 10 kilometres.

I say that I'm going to take part in the walk, but, of course,
that's the irony: I can't. But I'm at a place where I can accept
that I'm never going to be able to walk again with equanimity.
Unlike being unable to run, which cut me to the quick as a
teenager, losing my ability to walk has been largely untrau-
matic. I think I can say, hand on heart, that I'm OK with it.

Which, when you think about it, is not really surprising.
Though I was never told that one day I'd lose the ability to

walk (quite rightly), I suppose I was preparing for just this eventuality all my life, so I've had time to adapt to the reality.

I'm also conscious that I need to show Ellie that my wheelchair is my very best inanimate friend. Though it's by no means inevitable that she'll end up in a wheelchair (since CMT affects everyone in such markedly different ways), I'm also very aware that she knows that I am in one. Which means she probably does contemplate a possible future in one also (even if only for some of the time), in which case, it's really important she sees that it's not some dead weight or nuisance but an object that will give her freedom.

Preparing Ellie for this possible future is what the Waendel Walk is all about: to get her used to the positives, and show her that if being unable to walk does happen, it's not the end of the world. How much worse, I always think, to be walking around one day and then the next have that all taken away from you. That's what I always think about whenever I hear of people who've been in accidents and who suddenly find themselves quadriplegic or, even worse, tetraplegic. How enormous must the task of learning to function again seem to them?

* * *

We were blissfully happy, Lisa and I, when we got married. Once we'd (OK, I'd) got over the disappointment of not getting so much as a mouthful of our amazing double-choc wedding cake, it seemed nothing could pop our little bubble of happiness; we really did live in a world of our own.

Well, kind of. Where we actually lived was hardly paradise. Not by normal standards. We took up residence in a tiny purpose-built bedsit, one of a block of eight (four up, four down) that had been designed by a consortium of elves. The sort of place that you'd probably – no, definitely – steer clear of if you had a pet cat with a penchant for being swung around, but we didn't. Nevertheless in almost all ways it was delightful. The only downside was that it was only about a hundred yards from one of the runways at Heathrow Airport. Which meant that when the planes took off, Concorde particularly, we knew about it. Everything rattled: picture frames, ornaments, windows and doors, all our fillings ... But we didn't care. What was a bit of noise here and there between friends, when you'd managed to put a foot on the property ladder?

Work continued to be OK, if not riveting. Spurred on by my newfound positivity, I found the wherewithal to leave the YTS Training Centre, and got a new and interesting job at Northwick Park Hospital, working in occupational therapy. My role was to use computers to ascertain patients' cognitive skills after they had suffered a head trauma or stroke, which is perhaps why the word 'stroke' still has such serious connotations for me.

A year after being there, however, I was headhunted by a fulfilment company based in Hampton Court, and the extra income meant we could finally decommission our bedsit lifestyle (rather as British Airways decommissioned Concorde) and move into a much more practical two-bed maisonette.

There was a big reason to move. We'd always wanted children, ever since we first got married, and when Lisa told me she was pregnant, in the autumn of 1996, I couldn't have felt more excited. I remember sitting in church with her just a few days after we'd told friends and family, and how amazing it felt. Our bubble of happiness had just got even bigger.

It was a family service, in which children were particularly welcome. A large carpet had been spread out at the front of the church, on which the children would be invited to come and sit. Naturally, as children do, they all rushed up to sit down on it, and as they passed us, the grin on my face was so wide that Lisa laughed out loud, obviously having read my thoughts, and placed a hand on my arm.

'Don't worry,' she said, squeezing it. 'You'll be getting one of your own soon,' as if I'd been eyeing up a new car stereo.

And she wasn't way off the mark. Excited as I was at getting all the nursery paraphernalia, I was already looking into the future and making plans. Me being me, they were quite specific plans, involving the items I deemed most important. 'A giant train set' and 'Scalextric' were the top two, of course, though, sadly, I knew they'd have to wait a while.

Most importantly, we'd had 'the' conversation. (Though, in reality, it wasn't much of a conversation at all, and it certainly never occurred to us to seek any counselling; there was nothing a counsellor could tell us about CMT that we didn't already know – it's a very rare disease, after all.) We both wanted children and we knew what the risks were. We assumed there was a chance that our child would inherit the gene that might lead to Charcot-Marie-Tooth disease, though in reality we knew very little more. We couldn't, as there are so many variations of the condition, and even now they've not been able to identify which one I've got.

Of course we didn't want a disabled child – no parent would – but we didn't see the risk as being something that should stop us having a family. Why on earth would it? I only had to look in the mirror to answer that. Yes, I'd had my challenges while growing up, but I had loved my childhood and I also loved my adult life. I had an amazing wife, an enjoyable career, a brilliant family and fabulous friends. I could think of nothing – not a single thing – that would bring me up short and make me doubt that having children would be the right thing to do. My reasoning – and, thankfully, Lisa agreed with me – was that as I had the disease myself, I knew exactly what the reality was, so if we did have a child with it, I would be in the best place to support and guide that child in living with the challenges it might bring.

During Lisa's pregnancy we pretty much put it out of our minds. What's the point in stressing about something you can't change? And when Matthew came into the world, a robust and lusty 8-pounder, it couldn't have been further from my thoughts either. All I could think was: *I'm a dad! I'm a dad!* It was the most incredible feeling in the world. Of course we wouldn't know for some time whether the CMT gene had been passed on to him, but, again, we didn't need to know. What would be would be.

Besides, I was living very much in the present, for, ecstatic as I was to be a father to my little boy, I was becoming less of a mobile one by the day. There was no getting away from it: my condition was markedly worsening.

Lisa was still nursing then, working long hours at Hillingdon Hospital, while, having been made redundant when my employers lost a big contract, I'd become not only a first-time father but also a house husband. It was a struggle financially, but we coped, and I was actually having a fine time, as I could push Matthew in his buggy down to the local coffee bar every morning and read the newspaper while he had his nap. All well and good – the buggy was another crutch to lean on, another way to convince myself that, while I needed a wheelchair much of the time, I could still get about on two legs.

But as Matthew grew and increasingly didn't want or need a buggy, my crutch vanished. Soon I realized that while I could still walk to the car, I could no longer walk to the corner shop, and I was starting to need the chair more and more.

Then one day I couldn't even manage to get to the car. We were about to go into town when my knee suddenly gave way, and I badly tore one of my cruciate ligaments. I don't think I have ever known pain like it. And as if that wasn't bad enough, I had to undergo a procedure in hospital to evacuate the bleeding inside the knee. So it was a double whammy that day; intense pain and terror, for the needle they used was frankly huge.

Now I knew I had to accept that I had taken a dive. A nose-dive. This disability of mine was definitely getting worse.

Still, we limped on. In my case literally. And there were positives. I'd been doing some private work to help the finances, which would stand me in good stead for the future, and having had the time out to focus on the important things in life, at the end of that year I landed a new job.

And our family grew when, in 1999, Lisa gave birth to Amy, and we settled into a new life in Wellingborough. After the maisonette, our four-bed detached house felt like a mansion. There was only one major issue: it had stairs.

I think it was around then that the relentless nature of CMT properly began to sink in. Yes, I could manage the stairs, but I had to manage them rather creatively, crawling up them every time I wanted to go upstairs and coming down on my backside, like a toddler.

No matter, I thought. I will get a stair lift installed. And though it was a ready target for cheap jokes, much like meals on wheels and Saga holidays, I didn't see the lift as a defeat. I saw it as giving me a new freedom; it gave me the opportunity to continue living life independently.

But I was all too soon reminded that my independence could be illusory. One night I wanted a glass of water in the small hours, so I decided to go downstairs and get one. I folded the chair-lift seat down at the top of the stairs, as per usual, but, perhaps because it was dark and I was disorientated, I lost my balance. I fell down the stairs, from the top to the bottom, bashing just about every part of my body on the way down.

With all the breath punched from my lungs, I lay at the bottom, stunned, trying to work out what the heck had just happened. And, more importantly, what *would* happen. I tentatively tried to move, but soon realized it would be impossible. My back and hip really hurt, as did – more worryingly – my head, which I knew I'd hit hard. Which left me in something of a predicament. Lisa was on night shifts, so I was alone with the children and had no alternative but to yell upstairs and try to rouse Matthew, who at that time was just seven years old.

It all worked out – Matt was able to rouse the next-door neighbour, who called an ambulance – but the whole episode left me shaken and upset. What if such a thing happened again? What if something worse had happened? I think what shook me most was the thought of what *could* have happened: how badly I could have been injured – and with two sleeping children upstairs, as well. I'd been lucky. In fact I had been incredibly lucky. What if I wasn't so lucky next time?

My luck was certainly running out at work. My falls there had gradually gone from being occasional unfortunate occurrences to being so frequent that I no longer had to write them up in the firm's 'Accidents at Work' book. No, as well as quipping that I should have a season ticket for every hospital up and down the country, now they had furnished me with my very own book.

Though the pressure to stop trying to walk was subtle, I knew it was there, from both my employers and my own nagging conscience. Constantly falling, and getting injured, was inconveniencing everyone, not to mention risking a serious leg or head injury. And I was a father; I had a responsibility to my children not to blight their childhoods by getting seriously hurt

The only problem was that accepting the inevitable was so depressing. Though using my wheelchair more would obviously keep me safer and rest my leg muscles, not walking would just as surely cause them to weaken, causing my chances of ever walking to ebb away.

For the first time since I'd been so grateful to have God enter my life, I felt a sense of irritation. Couldn't he just give me *one* break?

MAY

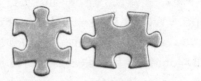

2 May 2012

Number of tickets in my hot sweaty hands for a recording of
*   BBC's Top Gear: 3.*
Which means ... number of challenges now completed:
*   A deeply gratifying 9.*

I am going to *Top Gear*. I am going to *Top Gear*. I am GOING
TO *TOP GEAR*!!!! It's official. I am going to see a live recording of *Top Gear*, when they next begin recording, in February
2013. And I have two extra tickets available, for the most
deserving, naturally. I see great potential in this state of
affairs ...

11 May 2012

Number of Waendel Walks completed today: 1.
Number of hours I spent training for it: 0. Well, compared to
*   the half marathon, it would be a walk in the park, surely?*

That's what I thought. Well, initially I did. And why wouldn't I? When I added taking part in the Waendel Walk to my list of challenges I had only one aim in mind – to be a part of it: to enjoy a push around my home town, meet new people and have fun. Which I appreciate doesn't make it sound terrifically challenging, much less 'extreme', but, to be fair to me, it wasn't on my extreme list.

Training for the half marathon, however, had quickly put me straight. Though at just 5 kilometres (or 3 miles) the walk – the shorter of the two walks in the event, around the environs of Wellingborough – would be a fraction of the distance of the half marathon, my training for the half marathon revealed one important caveat: Wellingborough is not only hilly but also full of potholes and damaged pavements. And when I did the Waendel Walk these turned out to be every bit as cruel and unforgiving as your average Saxon warlord, any day.

Still, I got round, and didn't break any fingers, though the fun aspect, it has to be said, felt distinctly lacking. Hard to feel you're having fun when you're trying to fit in with a bunch of walkers. Being wheely challenged, they all go so slowly, and for a veteran of the Adidas Silverstone half marathon, it was seriously hard to keep from ploughing into them all the time.

But there was at least one fun element: my camera. Ian Blackett, who walked with me, set me up with one of his funky photographic gismos, which he set to take a picture of the walk every five seconds, from its perch at the top of a pole above my head. It made my wheelchair look a little like a bumper car, which felt appropriate, particularly when he

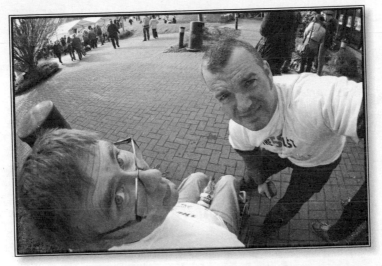

Ian Blackett and me getting set to start the Waendel Walk.

created a film from the footage – speeded up, it looked like
something off *The Benny Hill Show*.

Not that I was striving for comedy; far from it – I was striving for home and dinner. Oh, and wine. Oh, and the camera,
if you're interested, is called a GoPro Hero, and is widely available. Just wish the hero sitting underneath it (and note the
all-important knee-toning bottle of water) looked ever so
slightly more heroic …

17 May 2012

Halfway round-up!
Number of challenges now completed: A nice and not-bad-at-
all (given the killer winter) 10-plus-a-good-bit-of-
the-jigsaw.
Number of challenges marked 'ongoing' actually going, in the
'on' sense: Another supremely satisfactory 7.

It seems incredible that, in birthday terms, I'm now over half-way through my year. It's also good that, give or take a few ongoing challenges, I'm at least a third of the way through The 50 List as well. Cutting to the chase, though, I am a little behind. Not that I expected otherwise – not when all that snow fell, particularly – but it's already May, and before I know it, it'll be 'the run-up to Christmas'. That starts in about July these days, doesn't it?

I know I can do it. That's the key thing. I have belief in myself. And I'm so grateful that I've always had that cup-full mentality, because without it, it would really be so easy to give up. In some ways, it's actually better that I'm playing catch-up, because what will Ellie learn from me if it all seems too easy? I want her to watch me *live* the challenge, to see I *am* challenged, that it's difficult, because what I want her to learn above all from this is resilience. Resilience and the sort of self-belief my parents fostered in me. I want her to learn not to give up, however tough the going gets, because I know that for her, in comparison with her peers, it's going to be tougher in so many ways.

'So what's next?' Mattie wants to know, as he peers over my shoulder. It's early evening, the weather's warm, the sun is still just in the sky. We're sitting in the conservatory, making the plan for the second half, while Ellie sits and reads and Amy catches up with some homework.

'Let me see,' I say. '"Make a clay pot" … "Learn to wood turn" … "Get one of my photos printed in a national newspaper" …'

Matt shakes his head. 'No, I mean, like, *proper* challenges.'

I give him my indignant look. 'What on earth do you mean? They're all proper challenges!'

'No,' he says. 'I mean as in *exciting* ones.'

Well, I'm not ruling out a frisson of excitement during the wood turning; there's that all-important scope for losing a finger, after all. But Matt won't see that, of course. He's a teenage boy, after all.

'OK,' I say. 'Let me see …' I cast my eye down the list. 'Rockingham,' I say, pointing to it. 'Next week, racing an S60 Volvo round the circuit. Then there's Santa Pod, of course –'

I watch his eyes light up. 'Course. I'd forgotten that. What is it you're doing at Santa Pod?'

'I'm going to ride in the twin-seat dragster, remember? Well, allegedly.' This is more like it, I know. This is proper boy stuff. Fast cars. *Very* fast cars.

'Is that the long one?' he asks. 'The one with the big wheels at the back?'

I nod. 'And the small wheels at the front. Indeed it is. No 0–60 here, though – it goes 0–160. In about eight seconds flat. Can you imagine that? I can't wait.'

Ellie looks up at us. 'How fast is that?' she asks, though I suspect out of politeness rather than because she wants to know.

'Fast,' I tell her. 'Super fast. Much, much faster than our car can go. Almost twice as fast as our car can go, in fact.' I make a whoosh sound and shoot my arm forwards to illustrate. 'Really, *really* fast.'

'Really, *really* fast,' agrees Matt. 'REALLY fast.'

Ellie takes this on board, nodding sagely, as if computing relative velocities as we speak. Then she shakes her head.

'Yes,' she says. 'But why the *rush*?'

We go on then, Mattie and I, over our evening meal, to try to convey, in that way only enthusiastic males can, just 'why the rush' when it comes to experiencing speed. 'To feel the experience of G-force as the car launches,' I tell her. 'To feel the power of that enormous engine and then the negative G-force when the parachute is released.'

This throws some confusion into the mix. 'Why do you need a parachute?' she asks, perplexed now. 'It's not as if you're jumping out of a plane.'

'Not Dad,' Matt explains. 'It's the car that has the parachute. So that it can slow down really quickly, as going at that speed it would go right through the boundary fence.'

'But if it didn't go so fast,' Ellie begins, 'it wouldn't need one, would it?'

Perhaps drag racing isn't going to be her thing.

No, Ellie's thing, this particular evening, since we're getting our head round challenges, is to tackle one of her favourites in the 'ongoing' section: 'Play more board games'. Ellie loves playing board games, and adding this to The 50 List was an easy decision for me in any case since the night a few months earlier when we were all sitting down after dinner and it occurred to me that every one of us (yup, I'm as guilty as the next man) was locked in conversation with our electronic devices rather than each other. Kids on iPods and Nintendos, Lisa on her iPhone, and me doing a terrifically important something on my trusty iPad.

So now we're playing games regularly, and it's been great. And not just for the brownie points, either. It has another important fringe benefit: it also constitutes a night off from the flipping jigsaw. So while Lisa and the older two and I clear away the dinner things and load the dishwasher, it's up to Ellie to make tonight's selection.

'Trivial Pursuit,' she announces, as we reconvene around the dining table. Which suits me fine. I'm pretty good at Trivial Pursuit.

'I think I won last time, didn't I?' I say nonchalantly as I pull up my wheelchair. I am all about the business of it being about the taking part rather than the winning, but at the same time I'm fiercely competitive. Though it's only a game, as I'm always fond of telling them, there's none of this 'letting them win on purpose' lark with me.

'You won't win this time,' Amy tells me, pushing the box lid across the table. And she's right. There's no danger. They'll all beat me – including Lisa.

Disney Trivial Pursuit, to give Ellie's choice its full title. Dammit. Outnumbered and outgunned.

*   *   *

Faith in oneself is one thing; faith in God, quite another. If completely losing the use of both my legs gave me cause to doubt my faith as I hit my thirties, then, with the birth of our third child, it was really tested.

Not that we were anxious when Lisa found out she was pregnant with Ellie. On the contrary. Like any other young couple, we had plenty of energy, and couldn't have been more thrilled at the thought of a new addition to our little family. And after two trouble-free births, there was nothing to suggest that the delivery of our second daughter would be anything other than straightforward. But little Ellie didn't seem to want to come out. Time and again Lisa's contractions kept strengthening and then subsiding, and she was given a drug to help maintain them. Unfortunately, however, the tourniquet that had been used when setting up the drip hadn't been removed, so that when it was finally noticed, a big slug of the drug hit Lisa's bloodstream, resulting in a contraction that lasted three or four minutes.

Ellie arrived safely soon afterwards, but that huge contraction scared me. Was it an omen? No, of course not. Just a simple oversight; one of those things. Lisa was fine. Ellie was fine. That was all that mattered. And though our concern for Ellie increased when her learning difficulties were diagnosed, CMT couldn't have been further from our minds. Again, what would be would be.

Ellie's diagnosis came at around the same time mine had. She was in the reception class at school when Lisa and I first made the leap from wondering 'if' to amassing evidence for what we already knew, deep down, to be true.

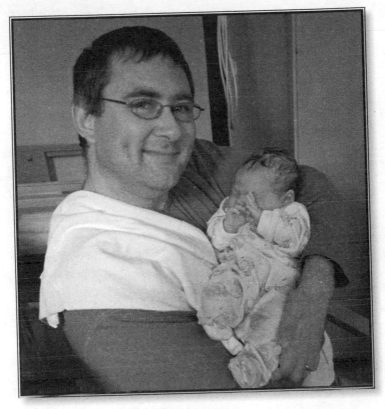

Proud dad with baby Ellie.

It had begun when Ellie was a toddler. Whereas Mattie and Amy had always been chomping at the bit to be out of their pushchairs, with Ellie it had been different: she was much happier to sit down, and if she did begin walking anywhere, it was always slowly, as she tired very easily. Consequently, once she was walking full time, it took a long time to get anywhere, even just walking to school and back.

On family outings it became even more evident. Where her siblings had boundless energy if we went somewhere, like the zoo, Ellie would be constantly begging to be allowed on my lap. So much so that one of my standing jokes of the time was that I had become the family wheelbarrow.

As had been the case with me, Ellie's gait wasn't quite right, and her teachers began reporting other concerns to us, telling us that she tended to tire easily, and would have difficulty getting off the floor again after storytime. They also noticed that she couldn't join in as well as her peers when they played any skipping and jumping games.

'We think she might have flat feet,' one of her teachers suggested. But Lisa and I knew that wasn't the problem. There was no way to sugar it; our worst fears had now been realized. So though we weren't as devastated as we might have been, since we'd always known this might happen, it was with heavy hearts that we took Ellie to see a doctor. And, though we didn't even need to hear it, after some initial non-invasive tests it was confirmed that Ellie did have CMT.

It was a dark time. Not so much for Lisa, who was and is so accepting and pragmatic. Which I suppose is how you'd expect her to be, under the circumstances. I guess she'd married me regardless of my CMT, embarked on having children with her eyes open, and had had years of exposure to a complex disability that hadn't blighted our lives. But our mothers, in particular, were devastated. Though it had never been discussed at the time, Lisa's mum had just assumed we'd never have children, and now we'd gone and 'pushed our luck', having a third child when we already had two healthy little ones, she felt we'd been very reckless indeed – why on earth had we taken that gamble? My mum was sad too; sad for Ellie, of course, but also for us, knowing from her own long experience how hard it can be to bring up a disabled child.

Me? Well, in truth, I was angry. Despite knowing it had always been a possibility, despite having discussed it and discussed it, it just felt so unfair of God to let this happen. Hadn't I been a decent person? Hadn't I risen to the challenges? Hadn't I done my best? What was the deal with a celestial score sheet that rewarded my years of effort and positivity by making little Ellie have to go through it as well?

It was one of the few times when I couldn't rationalize my feelings. We had both known CMT is very rare but also hereditary, but that didn't make the reality of Ellie having it any easier to bear. I guess I had just hoped that we might 'get away with it', and when we didn't, boy, was I angry with God. Angry, full stop. As was Matt – Matt especially. I remember that clearly.

Matt had his issues already. He was always such a good boy – he never really played up or behaved badly – but I knew, even if perhaps I'd subconsciously tried to bury it, that he had an underlying sadness about him. We didn't really discuss it, because I think he didn't want to upset me or make me feel guilty, but he'd communicate his frustrations to Lisa. It wasn't so much a rebellion as a kind of sad resignation that his dad wasn't like other dads. And I wasn't: I couldn't play football or go out on bike rides – couldn't even help with building his beloved Lego. So perhaps Ellie's diagnosis was really the tipping point. Whether it was or wasn't, he was desperately upset about his little sister's lot in life, and he found it hard to accept. He was angry at life, angry with God, and angry with us. All of which needed time and careful counselling. Perhaps it was in trying to help Matt through his anger that I was able to help myself cope with my own.

We hadn't got away with it, in short, and I had to deal with it. So the next step was to embrace it and help Ellie come to terms with it and live with it. For me – and I was so grateful that Lisa supported me – this meant no invasive and unnecessary tests. My parents had had no choice in the matter – they were dealing with something completely outside their experience, and had no choice but to take professional advice – but I was luckier. I knew exactly what we were dealing with and, more importantly, that this wasn't something that could be cured. So there was no point in Ellie becoming a pincushion, as I'd been, and having her childhood dominated by endless trips to hospitals.

For Ellie, we decided, it would be all about management. There was no need – and, to me, five years on, nothing's changed – to pinpoint exactly what type of CMT she had. It seemed much more important to deal with the symptoms. The best way to do that was to ensure that she saw a consultant neurologist who could manage her condition, with the right orthotics, physiotherapy and, unfortunately, corrective surgery.

But it seemed God hadn't finished testing me.

Yes, there was the nagging anxiety about what had happened with my vocal cords, and yes, Ellie's condition was obviously going to be a constant in our lives. But we were doing OK. We'd got through it, life was trundling on OK for us, and so when we moved house again, we did so with light hearts.

It was a good move. A positive time. A proper family time, too: we were moving because we'd decided to have Lisa's mum come to live with us. We were going to a larger house, a four-bed semi, with a big kitchen and conservatory, and plenty of space out front as well, to indulge my driving passions. It had ample space for all six of us *and* a number of cars, and we were naturally excited about creating what we knew would be our final family home.

Joan was a wonderful lady, and having been widowed six years back, was really looking forward to seeing out her time with us. As were we – particularly the children, who couldn't wait to have their loving gran on hand 24/7.

Only six months in, however, she was diagnosed with terminal cancer and told she didn't have more than a year to live. So be it, we thought. At least she's had a long and happy life. We'll just make the best of whatever time she has left. But within 12 weeks of being diagnosed she passed away, and Lisa was devastated. We all were. I was also angry. So where exactly *was* God while all this was happening? Did he even exist? It didn't really seem so.

'You'll bounce back,' I remember people telling me. 'Faith can be like that. People feel far from God sometimes, particularly when their faith takes a battering. You'll bounce back.' But I didn't. I was bouncing further away.

And I think what hit me hardest in terms of losing my faith completely was when, in May 2009, Lisa called me into the kitchen one day, as soon as I returned home from work.

I assumed it must be something church related – by now, Lisa was a lay pastoral minister. Or something to do with school, perhaps? Had something happened to one of the children? Whatever it was, her expression was serious. But not in a million years did I expect what came next.

'Nigel, your mum has died,' she said quietly.

Everyone's parents have to die. And my mum was 77 now, so she had attained a good age as well. I didn't have a 'get out of jail free' card in that regard; I knew that. The day was always coming. But why then? Why, when I hadn't had a chance to prepare myself and say goodbye to her? Why did I have to live with the knowledge that she died all alone, having collapsed on her kitchen floor, with no one to help her?

I broke down. I felt dizzy. I just couldn't take it in. It felt as though I was being deprived of air. It took me straight back to that night, when my mum had had to hold me as a terrified 20-year-old, as Lisa held onto me now, having just told me my father had gone.

Yes, a parent's death is an everyday tragedy, played out the world over – just as the birth of a child is an everyday miracle. But it's also a human tragedy, and I think that's what struck me most forcibly that day. Now I no longer doubted; I was convinced God didn't exist.

We gave Mum what we all hoped was a fine send-off.

The day after she died, I travelled to her house to be with my siblings, and the next day we took a train to London. We'd arranged to meet Derek, a retired vicar and friend of the family, in the hope that he would lead the service for us. His wife, Sybil, had been Mum's best friend since they'd been schoolgirls, and they had corresponded regularly all their lives. She had been a massive support to Mum after Dad died so young, and we knew having Derek and Sybil there would have been just what Mum wanted. He could perhaps, he suggested, even look over some of their correspondence as an aid as he prepared what he would say.

I was unprepared for how much that correspondence would touch me personally. I was a wreck at Mum's funeral, I don't mind admitting. From the minute I saw the coffin, I was off. So it was through tears that I sat and listened to Derek reading out one of Mum's letters. One that she had written to Sybil just after Dad had died.

As a child, and perhaps even as a young adult, free of big responsibilities, your parents so often just 'are', and so it was with me. I had had such a wonderful mum and dad – we all did – that hearing of my mother's emotional frailty at that time hit me almost physically as I listened to how she'd poured her heart out to her friend.

'I keep as busy as I am able to,' she'd written, 'in an attempt to fill the emptiness I still feel. But I have Nigel at home and I try to keep cheerful, for his sake …'

For my sake. To protect me from the anguish of seeing her heartbreak. It's OK, Mum. No need to worry about me any more. I'm doing fine. And I think – at least, I hope – I've made you and Dad proud.

25 May 2012

Number of challenges now fully completed: 11. Plus a load
  more ongoing.
However … number of times it has occurred to me that life in
  jigsaw-land would be so much simpler if all the wheels in
  all the steam engines in all the frigging world didn't look
  the same: 10 per minute squared.

Trains or cars? No contest, to my mind. That's not just because
they have fewer wheels. Nor is it because travelling by train if
you're in a wheelchair is one of the most difficult and dispirit-
ing things imaginable. No, it's cars every time because cars
can be driven. And sometimes not just any cars but race cars.

Being a motor-racing fanatic, I could sit and watch most
types of motorsport till there's a winner, however long that
takes, but I would always much rather take part. So when
there was an opportunity to add driving a race car round a
circuit to my list of challenges, I obviously jumped at the
chance.

Today was that day, and what a day it's been! I am buzzing
as I write this, and it's not because I'm parked up close to the
washing machine when it's on a spin cycle. It's because when
I'm driving round a race circuit, I feel so alive. Best of all, I was
able to forget all about my 'disability', as the car I was lucky
enough to drive – a Volvo S60, courtesy of a great guy called
Steve Collett – is one that can be adapted to suit the individual
driver. In my case, this meant I could brake using the hand
controls – something that made driving a great deal easier.

I couldn't race anyone else (this was a track day and as that meant members of the public would be involved, it had to be time trials only) but that didn't mean I couldn't race myself. In fact, in some ways, that was an even greater thrill because I was racing my own mind: fine-tuning my technique around the corners, improving both the entry and the exit, so that with each successive lap I could shave seconds off my time.

And I like to think I did OK; that if I were racing another driver, I'd hold my own. With a little more practice, at any rate. Definitely doing that again.

*   *   *

I suppose cars and racing have been in my blood since the first time I clapped eyes on Uncle Gerry's stock car. And when I was old enough and independent enough, I accompanied my aunt and uncle around the country, the trips becoming one of the highlights of the school holidays.

Uncle Gerry's car was driven by the team driver, Darkie Wright, who was and still is something of a stock car legend. The car was a bit of a legend, too. Stock cars are created from donor cars, often Fords or Fiats, but Darkie's drive was something of a superior breed, having the grill from an old Mercedes-Benz. It was revolutionary for its time, so I had the added frisson of being part of an elite clan, and sworn to secrecy in all things design related. This was because my uncle had come up with a clever way to make the walls of the tyres tougher. Punctures were a constant problem for all stock car drivers, because there was so much contact between the cars when they were racing. My uncle got around this by carefully cutting out the walls of old tyres and placing them round the inside of a new tyre to create a double wall. It was basic, but then aren't some of the best ideas the simplest? And it worked, leaving the other drivers constantly flummoxed about how the tyres on his car lasted so much longer than theirs.

By the time I was ten I was hooked. Not only on the whole business of racing; I also liked the lifestyle – the sounds and smells of racetracks, the people, the atmosphere of camaraderie and co-operation and the easy banter among the teams, which at the same time thrummed with competitive tension. You raced for only one reason: because you wanted to be a winner.

I also loved the feeling of being in that swanky modified coach. Sitting up high as it swung into whichever venue we'd arrived at, I felt like a king surveying his minions, and it was a feeling I really liked. Being in a racing team, looking at all the spectators looking at us – that was one of the best feelings in the world. It was as thrilling as I suspect it must have been to be in a circus at that moment when it rolls into town.

My uncle was extremely successful with his car, his team winning both the national and international championships. This meant he was allowed to paint the top of the car gold, so that he could let everyone know this was a world champion. Unlike in Formula 1, where the slowest cars start at the back, in stock car racing the slower and less experienced drivers start up front, meaning the fastest and best have to fight their way through them if they want to get to the front and keep winning. We had a new world champion now, too, in Pat Driscoll. As champion he'd have to pass every other car on the track in order to win, which made every race meeting even more thrilling. And, to my joy and excitement, invariably he did.

As I got older, I was introduced to other forms of motorsport. My brother Mark was a keen motorcyclist – still is, to this day – and used to have a number of friends who also had motorbikes and would often take me out on the back of them. One such trip was down to Brands Hatch in Kent to see some proper bike racing, and I remember being amazed at how fast the bikers took the corners. They leaned so far over it seemed that if they went so much as a fraction of an inch lower they'd touch the ground with their knee and come flying off. But for all the thrill of it, the gleaming bikes and the larger-than-life tattooed bikers, bike racing never really excited me as much as my beloved cars did. I would watch the rally cross or Formula 1 bike racing on the TV, but I preferred my live motorsport with four wheels.

For a teenager who spent much of his time on a trike or in a wheelchair, the thrill of speed – of being able to compete with those who had full use of all their faculties – made go-karting seem a natural thing to do as well. Though I never raced professionally, or continued as an adult (it was fun but incredibly tiring on the limbs), I would race my friends regularly. And it was this that may well have been the genesis of what would go on to become a lifelong passion for experiencing the thrill of speed myself.

It was definitely a passion. When Lisa and I decided to move to Wellingborough in Northamptonshire, it felt as if I'd died and gone to heaven. I hadn't realized at the time (well, perhaps subconsciously I might have) that I had relocated to the heart of motorsport country. As well as one of the stock car racetracks of my youth being only 40 minutes' drive away, Silverstone was just half an hour away. Then there was Rockingham raceway 20 minutes away – it was being constructed when we moved; and best of all, given my enthusiasm for extreme speed and drama, the world-famous Santa Pod, Europe's premier drag racing strip, was, and is, practically on our doorstep.

Where to start with just how thrilling I found my first visit to Santa Pod? If you're not into cars, I understand you might not get it but, if it's not too cheesy to quote a poet (in this case W. H. Davies), 'What is this life if, full of care,/ We have no time to stand and stare?' OK, so it *is* cheesy (even if the poem's not), but it also echoes my own philosophy. There's just so much to see in this short time we're on the planet, and I want to see everything I can.

And some experiences don't require you to be an 'enthusiast' in anything. Some things are just thrilling, full stop.

It was 2005 when I got my first thrill at Santa Pod. I asked my friend (and Amy's godfather) Dave Batchelor, who I didn't realize had already been there, if he fancied coming along with me to watch some drag racing.

'We should go and see a Top Fuel cars race,' he said, putting me straight on that point. He was obviously the expert here; I didn't even know what a Top Fuel car was. It was a May bank holiday when we went, and the whole place was buzzing.

So many people turn up to the big events at Santa Pod that what you first see as you approach is what appears to be an enormous campsite, as the adjacent fields are a sea of cars and tents and campervans. Once you've parked and headed down to the strip itself, you find yourself in a second sea, one of humanity, as families make their way not only to the grandstands but also to all the various food outlets, the pits or the funfair. There's always a funfair. Santa Pod is about cars, obviously, but it's also very family orientated, so there's something to suit every age there.

I was still walking at that time, though only just and with some difficulty, so it was something of a struggle to walk up to the grandstand seats my friend insisted we needed. In fact the bulk of it was achieved by a combination of hands and knees. But it was worth it. We really did have the best view in the house, looking down onto the start line and the two quarter-mile lanes, both of which we had an uninterrupted view of.

Drag racing is different from other kinds of racing, in that it's all over in a very, very short time. Consequently, a lot of the fun is in the preparation for the races, and the pits are all open to the public. Everyone gathers round; this is a place where spectators can get really close to the action and really see and hear everything that's going on. Then, once the race happens, it's all about acceleration. These cars have enormous power, and the format is always the same. Only two cars compete in each race.

I knew almost nothing else about drag racing that day, so I didn't have a clue what to expect, other than noise; Dave had advised me to buy some industrial ear defenders, and straight away I could see they were everywhere.

Noise was what I expected when the first two cars rolled out. They were muscle cars, the kind you used to see on

The Dukes of Hazzard: Dodge Chargers, Pontiacs, Mustangs and Chevys, all with big V8 engines and very little exhaust. And they delivered. They sounded like thunder – perhaps a cliché but in this case also true. As they revved up, it was almost as if you could see the air vibrating. Then, with an intimidating change in tone, which sounded as if several lions had all woken up at once, they were away, their front wheels leaping up as their drivers fought to keep control of them. They put me in mind of recently captured wild animals, straining at the leash to get away.

Seconds later, it was over, and the air was still once more. They'd just completed a full quarter-mile in ten seconds – twice as fast as the most powerful road car could go.

But watching the pairs of muscle cars do their thing was really just a warm-up for the next category, the main event, the one that we'd come along for: the Top Fuel dragsters. If I'd been impressed by the sight of the cars I'd seen so far, this was in a completely different league. It might sound melodramatic, but as I saw all these guys below us, pushing the first of these monsters into position, I really did feel all the hairs stand up on the back of my neck. They were simply enormous, and almost regal, it seemed – that was very much the sense I got – with their minions pushing them slowly and reverentially into place.

I might have had my mouth open, so awed was I by the spectacle. And the sheer size: just one of the rear tyres on these cars was wider than all of my car tyres put together – it really was that big.

And no wonder; these really were the kings of the drag world, guzzling nitro-methane to achieve dizzying speeds.

I couldn't have been more excited. Why had I never done this before? It was so incredible to contemplate that the fastest motorsport on earth was about to happen right in front of my eyes.

I watched one of the guys attaching a starter to the enormous engine, and as he did so I was aware of everyone either reaching for their ear defenders or, if they didn't have any, clamping their hands over their ears. As puffs of smoke from the exhaust began appearing, I realized how essential the protection was. If the sound of the muscle cars had felt like thunder, then this was like nothing I'd heard on earth, ever: a deep, crackling roar, which was violently, stupefyingly loud. So loud that I felt sure it could be heard for miles. It sounded angry, aggressive and terrifying, and as it rose in volume everyone automatically squeezed their ear defenders closer to their ears, me included.

What a spectacle! The cars in place, the crew chief motioned to the driver to roll forward; then came the burn-out, where the back wheels of the car begin spinning, not to move but to heat up the tyres to such a level that the rubber begins to melt, giving that vital grip. When an engine the size that these cars had transmits its enormous power to the axles, you've got to have grip or you'll go nowhere except straight up in smoke.

As the exhaust fumes started drifting, I could not only see them but smell and taste them. Nitro-methane has a sweetish taste initially; then I could feel it burning my nostrils. It was no surprise to learn that one of the by-products of nitro-methane is of a similar chemical composition to tear gas. Not that anyone seemed to mind. In fact some, I'd say, enjoyed it: I could actually see people sniffing the air to get a fix.

The burnout completed, it was down to the start line, and as the lights went green, signalling to the drivers that they could finally unleash their beasts, I realized that the Santa Pod publicity – 'Come feel the noise!' – was no hype. As the cars gripped and bucked and reached 100 mph in a single second, 'feel' was the operative word. Every fibre of my body, every sense, every molecule, was being assaulted by the raw, violent power of those incredible cars. I had never experienced anything like it.

It took just five seconds for them to reach the quarter-mile, their parachutes exploding open. And just five seconds to hook me for life.

JUNE

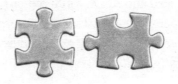

6 June 2012

Number of years since my first child was born: 15 exactly.
Number of inches he has grown in the last year:
  An astonishing 4!

To quote (or perhaps misquote) W. C. Fields, there comes a time in the affairs of man when he must take the bull by the tail and face the situation. Something like that, anyway. The main thing is that Mattie's 15 today and is now taller than me. You might think this is of no account, since I am now sedentary and no one need ever know this, but it is a milestone for a young man and an important one.

Matt and I have been lying on the floor to compare heights for quite a while now. I distinctly remember that there was a great deal of surreptitious shuffling around last year – all Matt's, of course – in an attempt to change the outcome, but this year, as we take up our usual spot on the conservatory carpet, there's not even a suggestion of a doubt about the reality. Matt is 5 foot 11 now – 3 inches taller than me. Of course,

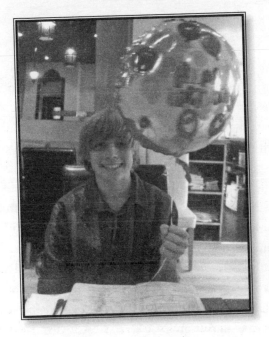

Matt's 15th birthday.

this is a very big deal to him. He's now officially the tallest member of the family; Lisa only comes up to his shoulder.

He is also maturing. Instead of going out for pizza, which has been a constant in Matt's birthday celebrations since he was knee high, his outing of choice is an Indian restaurant. Nevertheless, for all this new sophistication, he's still ridiculously pleased with the 'Happy Birthday' helium balloon we've arranged to have tied to his chair.

13 June 2012

Another week, another birthday – it's a very busy month, June. This time it's Amy's, though she won't be home to celebrate. Which is a shame, because it's a big one. Amy's 13; finally a teenager. But she's away on a school trip on the Isles of Scilly. And I'm sure she's having a great time, doing new things and meeting new people, so while we hate missing such a big milestone, it's a great opportunity for her and, in keeping with the independent young woman she's fast becoming, she's excited that she's going to spend her birthday away, with all her friends, and doesn't appear to be missing us one bit …

Not that Amy won't have some reminders of family and home. We've given her presents to her teacher so that she can be given them on the day, and, best of all, it turns out there's a brilliant cake maker on the island, so we're even able to whistle up a birthday cake for her, iced – if slightly luridly – in her favourite colour, purple.

'I'll be looking forward to tasting it,' I tell her when we call her to wish her a happy birthday. 'So make sure you bring us some back, won't you?'

She laughs. 'Not a chance,' she says. 'It's all gone. Every bit.'

Tsk. Just like our flipping wedding cake, all over again.

Taking a great photo – of a cake or otherwise – is a skill I've always aspired to, which is why getting one of mine into a national newspaper is on my list. It's not just a pipe dream; it's something I've been working towards for years now. Pretty much ever since that day when I saw my first drag race, and watched the Swedish photographer Stefan Bowman at work.

He carried three cameras and could switch lenses so incredibly quickly – something that seriously impressed me, as it would have taken me ages.

So my first trip to Santa Pod didn't just reignite my love of motorsport. It also began rekindling my passion for photography – something I'd worked hard at for a while in the 1980s. Back then, in the days of physical film, I was something of a keen amateur photographer, having caught the bug in 1981 when my sister Nicky worked at Moss the Chemists. It so happened that they sold cameras, and she was able to get me a discount – funny the way things lead on to different things, isn't it? I took to photography straight away, and though I didn't take it seriously, in the professional sense, I did learn to develop all my photos myself, which is a great way to learn how not to take a bad picture.

By 2005, however, we were in the digital age and, more importantly, my hand grip was much weaker. So I spent a lot of time trying to find a camera that would work for me, which is how I first met Ian Blackett. He patiently helped me make my selection. Given my specific needs – to be able to hold and use the camera easily – it took more time than it might have otherwise.

'What kind of photography do you want to do with it?' he asked as I weighed up different models (literally).

'I'm hoping to get a press pass for Santa Pod Raceway,' I told him. 'You might know of it. It's Europe's premier drag stri –'

Ian laughed. 'I do know of it,' he said. 'I'm their resident Run What Ya Brung photographer.'

Could a more fortuitous meeting have taken place? I doubt it. But what the hell was a Run What Ya Brung photographer when it was at home? I had no idea. So I asked him.

'Run What Ya Brung', he explained, 'is where members of the public can bring any car they want to the strip and then run it. I photograph them, basically. Anyway, maybe I can help you. Put a word in.'

True to his word, he did, putting in a word for me with the editor of a magazine called *American Car World*, who, just a few days later, helped me obtain my first press pass. It was a great day. Armed with my new digital camera, I was able to get pictures good enough to ensure I got passes to future events. My efforts paid off, and by the following Easter, I'd had three pictures published in the local paper and was beginning to see my work out there regularly.

As with so many apparently simple things, there was always the question in my mind about how long my fingers would hold out. But for the time being I was doing OK, and I was content enough with that. And not just because I was taking decent photos: because my press pass was about to become a passport as well, which would take me through a completely different door.

16 June 2012

Number of challenges completed after today:
    A comfortable-ish 13.
Number of patient wives deserving flowers and/or medals:
    Countless …
… Because number of Mazda MX-5 owners available for
    Saturday supermarket runs, lawn mowing, flat-pack furniture
    assembly or shelf putting-up: Hmm (just a guess, this one), 0.

Boys and their toys, eh? An exciting time ahead for me today, as I tick off one of the challenges that I've been most looking forward to since I came up with the idea of the list: 'Pay a visit to London's famous Ace Café'.

I say famous, but if you're not into cars and/or motorbikes, you might not have heard of it. Though if you are, particularly if you have a passion for classics, it's almost inconceivable that you won't have.

The Ace Café really is a legend in its own lifetime. Built back in 1938 to serve the traffic on the newly opened North Circular Road, it soon became a mecca, for bikers in particular, because of the fact that it was open for 24 hours a day – something almost unheard of back then. It became a service station, too. When both café and garage were flattened during a bombing raid on Willesden Railway Yard during the Second World War, that might well have been the last anyone saw of it. But such was its popularity, particularly in an optimistic post-war world, that the café was rebuilt and open for business once again only a few years later, in 1949.

As is echoed today in its styling, the 1950s and 1960s were the Ace Café's heyday. A favourite of ton-up boys and rockers, beloved by the newly christened 'teenagers', it soon became the place not only to see and be seen in but to go to admire machines, fix your own bikes and cars, swap stories and listen to rock and roll.

When it closed again at the end of the 1960s, to be replaced by a tyre workshop, it might well have gone the way of so much that was iconic in that period, and been consigned to history books and cherished memories. But there's no stopping a bunch of misty-eyed blokes when they get a plan going, and after a series of well-attended reunions in the 1990s, a plan was hatched to bring the Ace back to life. And that's what happened, to the great delight of petrol heads everywhere: it reopened in 1997. Since then it has gone from strength to strength, attracting not only the leather-clad clientele of its original heyday but also members of just about every cult car and bike club you can imagine, who flock there for its many special events. From Harley Davidsons to Hot Rods, BMWs to vintage Minis, if you rock up (to use the parlance) to an Ace Café gathering, you'll find yourself among friends.

Which is something of a roundabout way of owning up to the fact that I belong to the MX-5 Owners Club. And it's with six of my compadres that I'm travelling this morning, having met up in Northampton at stupid o'clock, in order to travel there in convoy down the M1.

For the uninitiated, there is something uniquely sociable about this sort of happening. Almost as soon as we're underway, we're joined by another London-bound convoy, and when we stop at the motorway services (not to eat, but to sweep through and collect others) our numbers swell to over 20 cars.

It feels great. The only downside is that I'm travelling alone. For all its loveliness, the MX-5 isn't the most practical of vehicles as, being a two-seater, it can accommodate only one passenger, and mine, of necessity, is my wheelchair.

But, once we've arrived, it's just about as sociable as it can be, and I spend as enjoyable a day as I've had in a long time, talking cars, and also cars, and, in between doing that, talking, erm, cars … the details of which I shan't bore you with.

I do my best not to bore Lisa with them either, once I'm home. A wife's patience only extends so far.

17 June 2012

Number of challenges complete: 14.
Though 13 would definitely have been more apt.

A sad day, as my Mustang (did I mention I owned a Mustang?) has finally been sold. I say 'finally' because it's been on eBay and in various classic car magazines for some time (hence selling it being one of my challenges) and I was beginning to think I'd never sell it. It was a fellow racer that bought it in the end.

Which is a good thing, of course, and in some ways I am happy to see the back of it. At least we now have a bit more space on the drive, and, more crucially, given our still precarious financial situation, it's provided some much-needed funds to help pay the mortgage.

But watching it being put on the back of a fancy trailer and driven away was still sad, and I miss it already. Not because it was fun to drive on road or race or track – though, boy, it was – and not because it looked good – though, undeniably, it did – but because it was my way to show people that I was capable of doing something outside the comfort zone: I was the only wheelchair-bound drag racer in the UK competing in the National Drag Racing Championships (up until 2010, anyway), so it's almost as though a piece of my personal success has gone along with it. Sentimental? Well, yes, maybe. But also true.

*   *   *

Given my track record as a teenager for doing wheelies, it would be no surprise to anyone, especially Lisa, that if there was a chance to actually cover the quarter, either in a drag car or in a dragster, I would be first in the queue. And the chance came in 2006, when Santa Pod put on its press day, when members of the press were given the opportunity to be passengers in a number of the different kinds of dragsters.

My first ride was with a driver called Nev Mottershead, who had a car that resembled a Toyota Supra, but only in the same way that a Scotch Bonnet chilli might resemble a small sweet red pepper. Under the bonnet there was a 9-litre V8 engine with 1000 brake horse power. Which meant no horse – however fleet of foot – nor pretty much any road car you could name, could ever hope to catch it.

I'd been trackside often by now, so was used to the phenomenal noise outside, but nothing could have prepared me for the intensity of the sound that engine made when I was inside; despite the full-face crash helmet, it was deafening. Nor could anything have prepared me for the experience of actually flying down the strip under such incredible acceleration; in fact, it's no lie that those nine seconds changed my life.

That, and something a fellow drag racer said to me when I got out. Her name was Carla Pitau, and what she said has always stayed with me, together with her enduring support. 'You only get one go in life,' she said. 'It's not a rehearsal.' And that was it. I was determined to make it happen.

To my relief – and enduring gratitude – Lisa was surprisingly supportive. Which was something I never took for granted. All motorsport is potentially dangerous – everybody knows that. And accidents do happen. I had witnessed some myself. But though they always looked terrifying, safety isn't taken lightly in such matters and there are lots of safeguards that ensure that 99 per cent of the time the driver walks away from an accident, unhurt. I think Lisa knew this, and perhaps also that in any case I wouldn't be deflected. At the time we met I was dabbling in gliding and go-karting, so she was well aware of my thrill-seeking gene. She also obviously knew how much this all meant to me and, to my delight, she even came along with me to view a muscle car that was for sale. Next thing she knew – well, by the end of that year anyway, which was as fast as I could make it happen – I had bought myself a 4.6-litre Mustang.

But it wasn't just a case of Lisa getting behind me. There was someone fairly important who needed convincing. Several someones, to be precise: if I wanted to race in the 2007

National Drag Racing Championships, then I needed to prove to the powers that ran it that I was safe enough to be given a competition licence.

Which, having got the bit between my teeth, I was determined to do. I sent in my application form to the Motor Sport Association and was invited to attend the medical advisory panel made up of doctors, motorsport consultants and other eminent medical personnel. It was something of a nerve-racking experience. Drag racing is a singular sport that requires a very precise skill, the art of it not being to drive the car in a straight line but to *keep* it in a straight line – which is way harder. When a car has the power of roughly five Formula 1 cars, it's a challenge to keep it pointing down the track.

The car I was going to race didn't have quite that much power, admittedly, but the principle still held. With my strength and dexterity issues, would I be safe? I knew I would be – I wouldn't have been applying to race otherwise – but I also understood they'd have concerns, and knew that meeting me, even though I could still walk a little, would do nothing to put their minds at rest.

One doctor got me to stand up and walk to the table, which I did – I had no choice – but I was very unstable. As I would be: I'd just driven a long way to reach their offices, and my legs were understandably quite stiff – something that was never going to be an issue in a drag race, of course.

I then had to demonstrate how good my grip was by squeezing the fingers of one of the doctors.

'His grip is weak,' the doctor said, as he observed how I was doing, immediately making my heart sink.

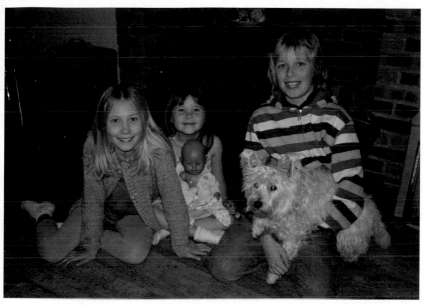

Amy, Ellie, Matthew and our puzzle-eating dog Berry.

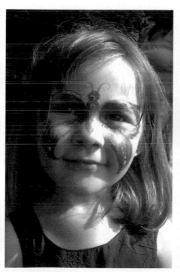

Ellie likes getting her face painted, opting for a butterfly this time instead of a tiger.

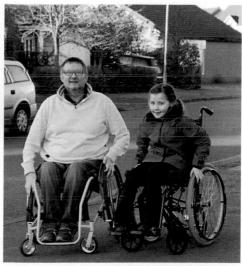

Me and Ellie. Ellie's chair was given to her shortly after the operation on her legs to help her get around.

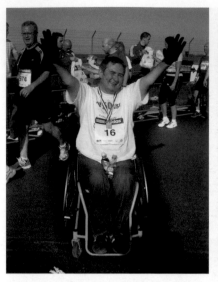

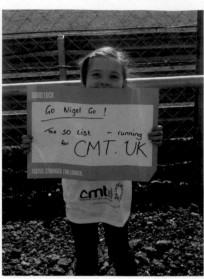

Just completed 13.5 miles and I'm surprised I can raise my arms!

Ellie, my number one supporter during the half marathon.

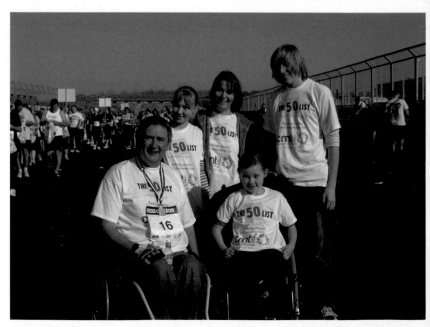

Me, Amy, Lisa, Matthew and Ellie, all wearing our 50 List/CMT T-shirts.

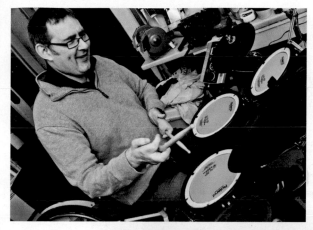

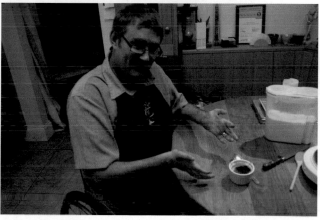

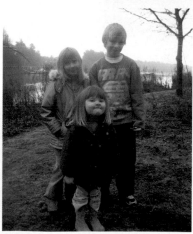

Top: It was good to get behind a drum kit again. Better still, it was an electronic kit, so I didn't disturb the neighbours.

Above: My first crème brûlée was divine! Etam Dedhar is an excellent tutor. I've made quite a few since and they have all turned out perfect!

Left: Amy, Matthew and Ellie on holiday. Ellie had just started showing signs of CMT at this time.

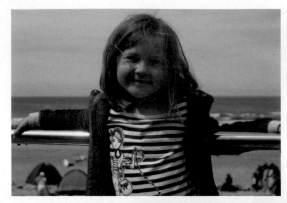

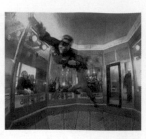

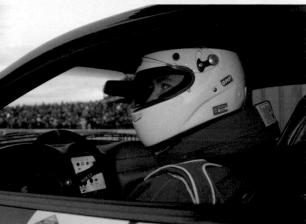

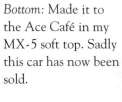

Top left: Ellie at the seaside in Cornwall. The one thing that Ellie loves to do is play in the sand.

Top right: Me during my indoor skydive challenge.

Left: Me sitting in my car waiting to race in round three of eliminations at Santa Pod Raceway.

Bottom: Made it to the Ace Café in my MX-5 soft top. Sadly this car has now been sold.

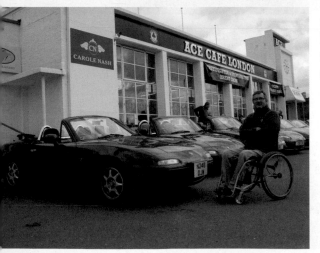

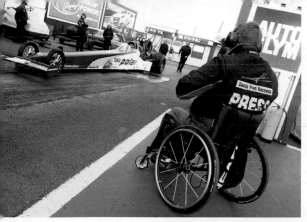

Covering Top Fuel drag racing at Santa Pod Raceway for our online magazine *Drag Racing Confidential*.

At the end of an amazing balloon flight: my family, the pilot Dave Groombridge, and Chris Pockett from Renishaw, who sponsored the balloon. This was a new wheelchair-accessible balloon and I was lucky enough to fly on its maiden voyage.

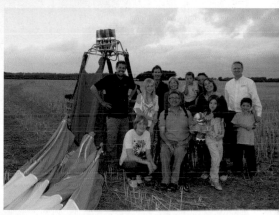

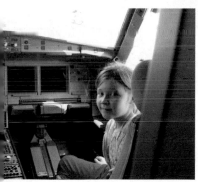

Ellie was very nervous when we flew to Italy so when we landed the stewardess invited her up to the cockpit. She was asked to flick the switch that turned everything off.

Matthew following my example. He had a go and he loved it. The rescue diver, who swam with him and his instructor, said he was a natural.

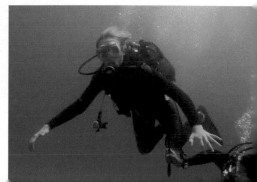

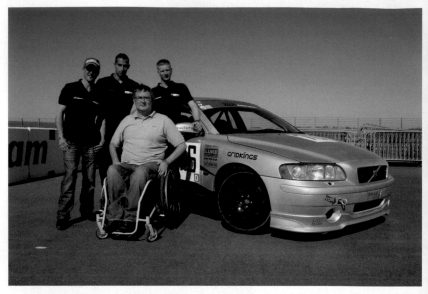

The need for speed. 'I can hear you smiling!' Paul Rivett, three-times Clio Cup Champion, said to me through the in-car intercom as I blasted through the chicane.

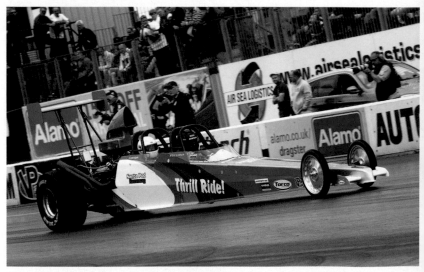

Steve Warner takes me for a Thrill Ride in the two-seat dragster at Santa Pod Raceway. This car can accelerate from 0–160mph in 8 seconds. What a rush!

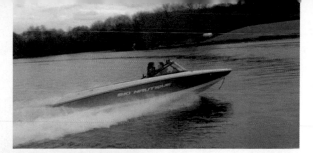

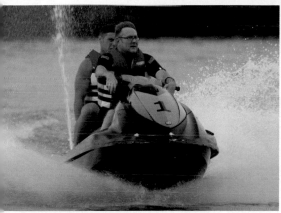

Top: The One Show arranged for me to be taken out in this powerboat and, boy, did it have a lot of power!

Top left: Getting the hang of the Jet Ski with my instructor, James, on the back enjoying the ride.

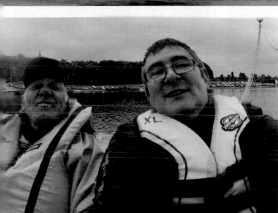

Left: Roy Child from Northamptonshire Sailability took me out in this accessible sailing boat and despite the day not being perfect we still had a great time.

Bottom: Me and Lisa at the Last Night of the Proms. An amazing experience. As you can see, I dressed for the occasion!

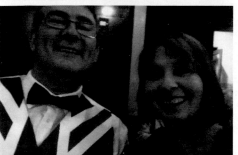

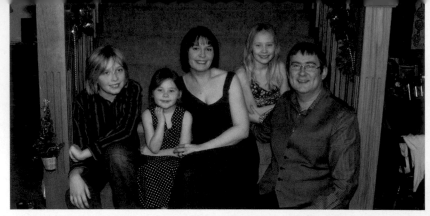

Matthew, Ellie, Lisa, Amy and me on New Year's Eve 2010.

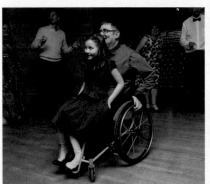

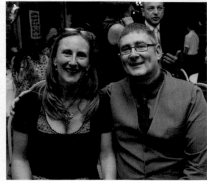

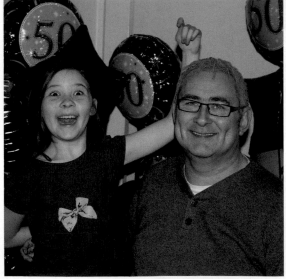

Above left: Me and Ellie on the dance floor strutting our stuff at my 50th birthday party.

Above right: My sister Nicola travelled all the way from California to be at the party.

Left: Ellie, over the moon that she got to make my hair pink, and she wants me to keep it this way. I don't think so!

'I have a racing steering wheel on my car,' I said. 'And I can grip that just fine.'

Happily, one of the panel members was David Butler, MBE, and he seemed to have knowledge of such things, because he immediately endorsed what I said.

But I still doubted they'd feel confident enough to pass me. I could tell by their expressions and general demeanour as the interview progressed. And my nerves weren't helping matters. As I left, it was with the conviction that this wasn't going to happen, until at the door it occurred to me that there was one thing I hadn't said, so I turned around. 'There's just one thing', I said, 'that I'd like to be taken into account. I should have highlighted the fact that I drove the 60 miles here with no problems.'

I have no idea whether it was that, or David Butler's confidence, but in what by then seemed like a miracle, it seemed I'd be able to race after all. He called me the next day with the astonishing news. 'You got your licence,' he said simply. I was away.

21 June 2012

Number of challenges complete after today's one: 15.
Thought for the day: Hmm. Now, where's my stock of flying
    vicar jokes?

Off to Airkix again today for some fun.

Not content just to have a go at skydiving myself, one of the challenges I've set myself is to get someone else to try it, and specifically someone with a 'disability'. After all, the whole thing is about inspiring those who have disabilities, so this felt like a natural extension. Choosing my 'victim', someone who might be interested enough to try it, was the work of half a second. It would be John Naudé, Ellie's godfather, who became priest of our church back in 2000 and soon a really good friend.

Whether or not he'd be up for it I wouldn't know until I called him.

'John,' I said. 'Nigel. Got a question to put to you. How do you feel about experiencing a free fall?'

John's been in a singular kind of job for a very long time now, so nothing fazes him. He gets asked all sorts of bizarre things. He didn't miss a beat. 'Hmm. Depends where I'd be landing, I suppose. Is this out of a plane?'

'No, but you'd still be reaching terminal velocity for two minutes.'

We're of a mind, the two of us. I knew this might tempt him. It did.

'How does that work?' he wanted to know. 'Without the plane part, I mean.'

I explained that on this occasion there was no need for me to toss him from a plane. He seemed almost disappointed.

'The plan', I said, 'is for me to take you to Airkix.'

'Ah, as you did earlier in the year. The skydiving. I remember now.'

'Exactly,' I said. 'And as one of my remaining challenges is to –'

John cut me off mid-sentence. 'I'll get my coat.'

*   *   *

So that was that, then. No encouragement necessary. And John enjoys his skydiving experience every bit as much as I did mine, which is going to be a surprise to no one. Because, like me, John doesn't see himself as disabled; he's just someone who happens to have a disability. In his case, it's spina bifida, but it's never stopped him doing anything, from being an active Church of England priest to being a great wheelchair basketball player and moving to Malawi – which he's doing in less than a couple of months from now, to help people less fortunate than himself.

When thinking about this challenge, I could have picked any number of people. I chose John, but equally it could have been Amy, who needs her glasses to see the blackboard, or my friend Mike Jackson, who's diabetic and needs insulin. But since, like me, John gets around using a wheelchair, he is more obviously 'disabled'. Which is what makes it such an inspiring thing to see.

Perhaps because I use a wheelchair myself, however, I don't see John as 'disabled'. I see a friend, a man with whom I have a great deal in common. I see a man who's up for anything, a man who shares my sense of humour, a man who shares my philosophy that life's there to be challenged. There's no sense of 'us and them', 'us' being the two of us in wheelchairs. I simply don't see the wheelchair at all.

Unfortunately, people so often do see the wheelchair, before they see anything else. I remember a few years back, when I was still trying to get around on two legs if I could, I was taken to hospital after one of my all-too-frequent tumbles at work. It was one of so many that I can only vaguely remember how and where the fall happened, and I'm not sure I can recall which hospital it was, either – it was just 'yet another spell in A&E'. But what I remember all too clearly is a conversation I had with a healthcare assistant while I was lying on the bed in a side room, waiting to be seen. I was in some pain at the time, the analgesics not having kicked in yet, so, to be fair to her, she probably caught me at something of a curmudgeonly moment. But the words we exchanged have stayed with me ever since.

She'd come in to replace my water jug with a fresh one, and, probably just keen to be friendly and make conversation, she commented on my wheelchair. 'Ooh,' she said, smiling. 'That's a fancy chair they've given you.'

'It's not a hospital chair,' I told her. 'It's mine.'

Her demeanour changed instantly, both in tone and expression. 'Oh,' she said. 'I didn't realize. I'm sorry.'

Which initially threw me. What on earth was she apologizing for? So it was my wheelchair – what of it? Why would she feel the need to say sorry? Did she think I might be offended that she'd been mistaken about who owned it?

I was just wondering how that could possibly offend anyone when she spoke again. 'Oh,' she said again. 'That's a shame.'

At which point I could have just let it wash over me, except I couldn't. Blame my irritability due to the throbbing ankle, or just call me plain old grumpy, but at that moment, I really couldn't let it go.

I sat up on the bed and fixed her on the end of a pointed stare. 'Have you ever played drums in a band?' I asked her.

She shook her head, looking confused. 'No. No, I haven't.'

'I have,' I said. 'How about water-skiing, maybe?' She shook her head again.

'I have. How about a go-kart? Ever raced in a go-kart?' Ditto. 'Swum in national competitions?'

Once again, she shook her head.

'So you've done none of those things?'

'No,' she said.

I smiled at her. 'That's a shame.'

Then I lay back down and closed my eyes again.

I don't know what the woman must have thought of me, but I felt it needed saying. She needed to be informed. Not to mention put in her place!

Of course, what she mostly needed to learn, looking back on that encounter, was to be careful to whom she spoke in those side rooms …

Discrimination takes many forms, of course, and not all of them are negative. But discrimination born out of a desire to do a good thing can still have a negative effect on the recipient. It may seem churlish to feel aggrieved when someone's only desire is to be helpful, but a little forethought goes a very long way in avoiding such an effect.

When I go into town, for example, to visit my local Costa Coffee, the entrance door is heavy, but I can manage it. So on the odd occasion when someone leaps up to help me without first checking if I need help, I feel niggled. It's not the help itself that niggles but the automatic assumption that help must be required. People often make such an instant connection: they see the wheelchair and they assume I must need assistance in some way. And while I'm grateful for the help (how could I not be? That would just be rude of me), I can't help but make a similarly automatic connection myself: that my independence has been taken away from me.

That is not to say I don't know when to ask for help – I do. If I'm injured, for instance, and in need of it, I'll holler. But human nature is human nature, and just as it's natural to want to help, it's also natural to want to hang on to your independence.

JULY

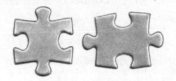

What we did on our holidays …

Our summer holiday this year has been more extravagant than any holiday we have had before. We normally go to places in the UK that are accessible, the only exception in recent years being Disneyland Paris, which was for the children's benefit rather than mine or Lisa's. In fact, the wheelchair and I spent most of our week there as Ellie's personal transport, and returned home with the bruises to prove it. But this year we've been lucky, and it's all thanks to The 50 List. When my friend Mark Harris offered me a trip to Italy to do one of my challenges ('Go scuba diving'), it would have been nigh on impossible not to turn it into our family holiday, as he suggested, especially since it meant I could also tick off another challenge at the same time: 'Swim in the sea after a gap of 30 years.' So that's exactly what we did.

I've known Mark since we were teenagers, having met him on a coach on the way to Wembley to see the Harlem Globetrotters – a trip arranged by the local church youth club. We soon became friends and would often go camping together, and it was on one such trip, down in Dorset with a load of other friends, that he introduced me to his gun. Mark was (and still is) an accomplished hunter, having bagged a number of wild boars, deer and other edible critters over the years, and when we were in Dorset he let me have a go at shooting as well.

'What, just like that? Is it allowed?' I asked. He assured me it was. We were camping in a farmer's field and Mark knew the farmer, so it was perfectly legal and safe. I don't think Mark is capable of being anything other than legal and safe, which is one reason why I trust him with my life in the water.

But that was Mark and this was me, and I'd never fired a shotgun before; and I was amused to see that he'd somewhat optimistically set up a cornflakes packet as a target a good 50 feet away. *Still, no harm in trying*, I thought, taking heed of Mark's instructions, taking aim carefully and pulling the trigger.

I'd opted to sit in my wheelchair to fire the gun, for reasons of balance (as in my lack of any) and, boy, was I glad that I did! Goodness only knows where I'd have ended up if I'd attempted to do it standing. As it was, once the gun discharged, I wasn't sitting in it any more. The cornflakes packet lived to be a target for another day and another marksman, and once the ringing in my ears had stopped and I'd scraped myself back up off the floor, Mark explained why it had all gone so wrong.

'You just didn't lean into it enough,' he said encouragingly. 'D'you want to try again?'

I didn't. I think both I and the good folk of Dorset would probably agree that was the sensible choice.

Visiting Mark in Italy didn't involve any encounters with firearms, but it certainly involved plenty of other encounters: with Italian food, Italian people and some breathtaking Italian scenery. Oh, and limoncello, which is just like my mum's lemon meringue pie, only served in a glass and containing alcohol. Which makes it pretty near perfect in every way.

And this was proper Italy, largely untouched by tourism. Mark's house is up in the mountains near the coast at San Remo, which is where my session of scuba diving was scheduled. We travelled there via a flight to Nice, which was something of an adventure in itself, because this was Ellie's first ever flight and she was frightened. While I was busy marvelling about how facilities for those in wheelchairs have come on in recent years, Ellie, who was once again using me as her personal form of transport, was getting more anxious by the minute. By the time we left the ground and got that familiar 'being pushed back into your seat' sensation, her grip on my hand was so strong she almost stopped the blood flow.

I'd tried to prepare her for what would happen, what she'd be hearing and what she'd be feeling, but fear is fear, and sometimes it can't be explained away.

But thank heavens for the cloud cover. It was an overcast day, dull and drizzly, and breaking into the sunshine above the cloud base worked like a charm. Suddenly all was well, because spread out just below us was an unbroken sea of fluffy white clouds. A bed of cotton wool, in fact, promising the illusion of a soft landing. Ellie beamed at me. 'I'm not scared any more, Daddy,' she said.

Sometimes an illusion is all you need.

Landing in Nice, it was so good to feel the sun on my face, and leave the drizzly British weather behind us. And what a first day our hosts arranged for us! On the way, we stopped at a local tavern, run by Mark's Italian friends Fabrizio and Graziella, and while Mark took Lisa and the children swimming down at the stream below the restaurant, I was happy to just sit on the veranda and look at the view. Sometimes doing nothing is the only thing to do. Beer in hand, sun on back – it was bliss.

After that, it was time for lunch – and that pleasing introduction to limoncello – before travelling the rest of the way to Mark's house and enjoying an equally beguiling evening, meeting Mark's friend Mike (who was also staying and was a great help throughout) and relaxing over another wonderful meal. Finally, once Lisa and the kids had gone to bed, we just sat there chatting, 3,000 feet above sea level – oh, the view! – and sipping liqueurs and brandy. What a day!

The following day, we hit the beach. The diving session Mark had arranged for me wasn't scheduled till the Monday, so over the next couple of days we took in the lovely beaches and relaxed. Ellie was happy to do just that – all she wanted was to play in the sand with Lisa – but Mattie and Amy were in the sea before we'd even unpacked our stuff. I very much wanted to join them, and it turned out I was lucky.

Sand and wheelchairs don't make the best companions ever, but they had an old wheelchair on the beach there, specifically for the purpose of getting the wheelchair-bound down into the water. That was me sorted, then. This was an opportunity I couldn't afford to miss, and within minutes,

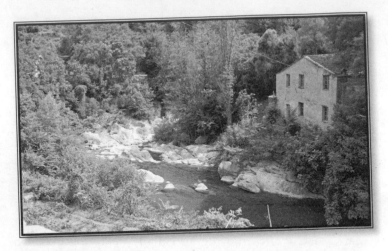

The kids had a great time swimming in the stream.

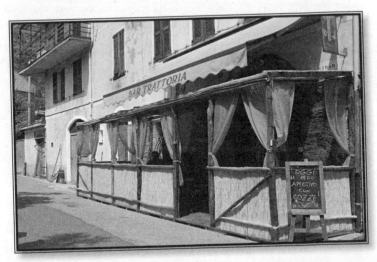

The Bar Trattoria – owned and run by Mark's friends Graziella and Fabrizio. We ate in this fantastic restaurant every day!

with the help of some obliging volunteers to push me down there, I was in the sea with the kids, and, boy, did it feel good! I was astounded by how warm it was: warmer than our local swimming pool – positively toasty. As I swam out of my depth, so that I couldn't feel the bottom, I felt as pleased as punch. This was definitely my idea of *la dolce vita*.

*   *   *

Being out of my depth and not being able to touch the sea floor is a big thing for me: it puts me on a physical par with other people; I'm not having to use my legs to stand, and nor are they, and I can swim as well as everyone else. It's like the skydiving, where the instructor and I became physical equals, and it's one of the reasons I'm so keen on Ellie swimming: that equality will give her such confidence. It's also wonderful to be able to do something so physical with Matt and Amy, just like any other father.

I've always loved swimming, ever since I was a small boy. My dad used to take us to the BEA club in Northolt, where he taught me and my siblings to swim and also dive. And it was in the water that I always felt most at home. 'You're more like a fish out of water than a fish out of water!' was something I remember Mum quipping to me often.

*   *   *

On the Saturday, there was a treat for the older kids as well as me. My own session of scuba diving had already been arranged for Monday afternoon, further down the coast, but in the meantime Mark, thinking the kids might fancy having a go too, surprised us by telling us he'd organized a session for them.

I went along with them. I didn't dive – it would have been unfair on my instructor, Vincenzo, since that had already been organized – but I was really just as happy to watch my kids doing something fun; like any parent, that's often how I get my kicks. And as Mark remarked later, Matt turned out to be a natural: he was suited up and sitting on the edge of the boat in no time, before plopping into the water backwards like a real pro. I was so proud.

Once Matt was in, it was time to prepare Amy. I could tell, even as she watched them put all the equipment on Mattie, that she was beginning to get a little nervous. I kept reassuring her as they prepared her, but in the end I could see tears in her eyes, so off it all came again, to her great relief. She didn't give up, though, and was soon persuaded to get into the water with just a regulator and goggles, so that she could at least get a sense of what it was like. And very soon she was swimming around with her instructor on the surface. I got in and joined her, and it was fun to be in the water with her, looking down and seeing Mattie far below us. I was just as proud of Amy as I was of him, because she had had a go: she got in and tried it out. Maybe next time she'll go to the bottom for a look around.

On the Monday afternoon, it was finally my turn to dive. Once again, I was taken out in a wheelchair, only this time it was a very clever sand-and-sea-going wheelchair, designed to go right into the water. Once I was kitted up with wet suit, air tanks, goggles, flippers and regulator, I was ready to roll – literally.

Sadly, though, compared to Matt's dive on the Saturday, it wasn't that thrilling. During the night there'd been a heavy downfall of rain in the mountains, and as we were diving right next to the river outlet that ran from it, we couldn't see a thing; I could only just make out Mark swimming in front of me. So in the end we had to call it a day.

But though it was disappointing not to be able to get to the seabed as Mattie had, I definitely got a taste for scuba diving. And at least it was another item ticked off the list. And with an invite to go back again in my metaphorical pocket, I'm not *too* disappointed. Same time next year …

14 July 2012

Number of challenges now completed: 17.
Number of years since Lisa gave birth to our third child:
    A perfect 10.

Ellie is ten years old today, which prompts the usual parental reflection on how ten years can disappear in such a short space of time. I know that's a step on the road to becoming the sort of elderly relative who pats children on the head saying 'My, haven't you grown', but, really, where *did* that time go? Was it a whole decade ago that Lisa and I were bracing ourselves for another year of sleepless nights? Ten whole years since we last began changing nappies?

*   *   *

It's been quite a ride with Ellie, for sure. But, happily, a smoother ride than perhaps Lisa and I had feared. We've had our bumps along the way, but that's part of parenting anyway, and Ellie copes with her CMT very well. She's been remarkably accepting as she's grown and begun to understand what it means for her. She did once ask us why she had CMT and her brother and sister didn't, which we could only answer honestly: we didn't know. But since then she's been incredible. She's just got on with it.

The biggest milestone in her young life has obviously been her surgery in 2010, which, for Lisa and me at least, was very stressful. It was major surgery, too, to correct a problem with her gait: because of her CMT, both her feet were beginning to turn in. It was a procedure called a tendon transfer, and it worked very well; they took a healthy tendon and moved it on both legs to compensate for the muscle wastage that was happening, and it restored her feet to an almost normal position – though this will need looking at again in the future. Ellie was a trouper; throughout it all, she never once moaned, and I think that says it all. I like to think she's inherited some of my 'Sod it, let's just get on with it' attitude. Well, so far ...

* * *

Ellie's tenth birthday celebrations began yesterday (well, she's a girl), and in what now seems to be the accepted fashion for young ladies *d'un certain âge* she requested and was granted a sleepover. She had three friends over, and the party began mid-afternoon, when they took over the conservatory (manfully supervised by Amy) for what I'm reliably informed was a mass 'makeover'. I say 'informed' because, being a man, I steered well clear. They then moved on to the cinema (well, the living room anyway, accessorized with crisps and popcorn), where we allowed them to camp for the night (we're not stupid – it's the furthest place in the house from our bedroom).

That done, today's family celebrations were more of an after-show party. We had a family lunch at the local pub, followed by an evening indoors, comprising – and there's a theme building here, if you look hard – *The Princess and the Frog* on DVD, crisps, Coke and popcorn …

15 July 2012

Number of weeks I've been looking forward to today's
    challenge: Lots.
Number of miles per hour you can get to in 8.12 seconds:
    158.5. Wow!*
Number of petrolheads who'll be green with envy reading that:
    Too numerous to mention …*

There's a saying in drag-racing circles: that if your ambition in life is to be a millionaire drag racer, then you have to start out as a multimillionaire drag racer.

In short, drag racing is expensive. It is also addictive. As my mate Vic Amato says, 'Going fast is fun, and you can never have too much fun.' He's absolutely right. As any drag racer you meet will tell you (him included), once you've gone seriously fast you always want to go faster; it's that kind of push-it-to-the-limit sport. But for every extra mph, you need increasingly deeper pockets, which is why the partners of drag racers everywhere have my deepest sympathies …

Anyway, the point is, I went to Santa Pod and was driven along the strip very, very fast. Amazing. Fantastic. The end.

18 July 2012

Jigsaw status update: Grrr.

In choosing 'important steam locomotives and their inventors', I fear my choice of subject matter has been slightly ill judged. Yes, Ellie's keen to help, but that is becoming far more 'in theory' than 'in practice' now. And I suppose I can't blame her. Although I am a man and have a well-developed male interest in things that are made by men and go fast, even I am beginning to become sick of the sight of all these portly chaps and their even portlier engines. Yes, there has been some progress – yesterday, for instance, I managed to complete a whole section of boiler on a green train – but such is my sense of ennui that I haven't a clue what the train is called; I know nothing other than it's green and it's a train. That's kind of how it's getting for me now.

This morning, I was whiling away an hour looking for a piece with a picture of a guy's head on it, and as I dredged the box lid, even the singular sound of massed jigsaw pieces in a box lid was beginning to grate. I've given up on the whole history-of-steam-engines malarkey now. All I want is to get the blooming thing finished. Not least because as I picked up a piece that, at first sight, looked as if it might be the one, I feared imminent mutiny.

And when I picked up another, and saw what was on it, I realized there were pieces in my box lid that should not have been there. Last time I checked, there was no note in engineering history that put Tinkerbell centre stage in development. But this was no surprise, really, because a few days back, in an attempt to stick to the spirit (if not the letter) of the law regarding our shared jigsaw endeavour, Ellie had arrived at the coffee table and started setting up one of her Disney jigsaw puzzles at the other end of it. Note to self: be of stout heart. And reclaim the flipping table.

But the day got better. Where putting together a jigsaw has been a long-term activity to test both my manual dexterity and my patience, the activity I deserted Tinkerbell for, though still a challenge for my hands, is pure therapy. I've always rather fancied having a go at making some pottery, because the idea of making something out of raw materials – of taking a lump of clay and using what little strength I have in my hands to fashion something that can be used, looked at and admired – appeals to me. There was never a defining moment when I thought to myself: *Yes! I'd like to try that!* It was just something I always fancied doing. Though I should point out – and already have, to various people – that watching Demi Moore and Patrick Swayze in a certain scene in *Ghost* has absolutely nothing to do with it.

I make my pot today courtesy of a guy called Rob Bibby, who runs Rob Bibby Ceramics, a pottery centre about 45 minutes' drive away from where I live. He's really welcoming and gets me stuck in at the wheel in no time. He's also gracious enough to comment, as I produce my first pot, that for a beginner's first attempt it's pretty good. It has straight lines, at least, and most importantly, no wobbles – I was firm with Lisa: she was not to get behind me and mess things up.

But, as is often the case, my impressive dexterity as a beginner soon wanes. As the second, third and fourth pots all wobblingly testify, it was just that other thing beginners have: luck.

No matter, though. The potter's wheel is definitely great for inner calm. I am ready to do battle with the jigsaw once again …

AUGUST

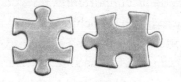

15 August 2012

Number of capital cities visited so far: 1 – Edinburgh. Finally.
Number of double single malt whiskies needed to be imbibed
 to be officially declared drunk in charge of a wheelchair
 (or indeed, to be able to say that): 4.

What a city! So. Let me see. What exactly did I do in Edinburgh? Yes. According to the notes I have before me on my iPad, my brother Gary and I definitely went to Edinburgh.

I'm lucky: I've always got on brilliantly with my siblings, and their support and encouragement this year – well, for all my life, actually – has been incredible. You take siblings for granted when growing up – your brothers and sister are just 'there' – but when I look back, I realize just how amazing they were. I never felt that my CMT made any difference for them – not in a bad way. And, crucially, they didn't treat me with kid gloves. I well remember how I'd ask my brothers if I could go out on some adventure with them, and one or other of them would say, 'Yes, but first go upstairs and get yourself a jumper.' And then, of course, I'd come down and they'd be gone. But last time I checked, this would seem to be regular big-brother behaviour. Big brothers don't want little brothers cramping their style, and more fool me for not thinking that generally, in midsummer, you don't need a jumper to go out to play.

I'm glad Matt and Amy have the same relationship with Ellie. Like my own siblings, they support her but don't mollycoddle her. It's particularly good to watch how Matt – who had such problems coming to terms with things – now treats Ellie just the same as he does Amy. Yes, they have their spats, but what kids don't? That's normal and healthy. We wouldn't want it any other way.

Gary and I had the odd spat as youngsters as well, but after Dad died, he was a great older brother to have around: on hand not only to help with advice but also to put me straight when, as a rather cocky 20-something, I got a little out of line from time to time. We also share the same sense of humour, so to hit Edinburgh right in the middle of the festival (him via a plane from Germany, me via a train from Peterborough) was pretty perfect timing.

It was also perfect in another respect: since one of the items on my list is 'Write a comedy sketch', it gave me a perfect opportunity to grab both tips and perhaps material at the Fringe. Or, rather, would have given me, were I able to recall any of the finer details. I can't, as one of the other things we did was visit Glengoyne Distillery, and as Gary was driving, I had to do the decent thing, obviously, and do a double round of tasting on his behalf.

23 August 2012

Va-va-vooooom!

My mate Vic Amato's maxim that going fast is fun and you can never have too much fun – which he has written on his race car – explains the inclusion in my list of today's challenge. I've never ridden a motorbike – though never say never! – but riding a Jet Ski is the closest thing to riding a motorbike I can imagine, the only difference being that you do it on water.

Once again I am indebted to kind friends. In this case it's the folks at Lagoona Park in Reading, where I did it. Shirley and her son James couldn't have been kinder or more helpful, allowing me to blast around their lake, free of charge, for as long as I wanted, just so that I could get this one ticked off the list.

29 August 2012

Into each life, a little rain must fall … Or, as I believe they say,
*   'Croeso y Cymru!'*

It would be nice to be able to say that every item on The 50 List was special – enjoyable, unforgettable and 'I want to do it again!' compelling (see entry above) – but alas Cardiff, the second of my capital cities list items, evoked no such feelings. The day started badly, and, as often happens when you get off on the wrong foot, it went mostly downhill from there.

We were a two-man team for our overnighter – me and Mattie, to be precise – both with our own reasons for visiting the Welsh capital. In my case, it was as part of my quest to get the full set for the list, obviously, but also because I'd heard so much about the city over the years and wanted to take a look at the stunning architecture I'd read about. Matt's reason was straightforward: to immerse himself in all things *Doctor Who*-ish, the modern series having been filmed in the capital, which also houses a *Doctor Who* exhibition.

We decided to drive, given that train travel looked like being complicated and expensive. This meant our first job on arrival was to find somewhere to park the car, our city-centre hotel being all out of disabled parking spaces. It took 40 minutes to park, and, as a bonus, we were expected to pay a king's ransom for the privilege, which naturally didn't put me in a good mood.

And it was a mood that was unimproved once we'd finally checked in and our ordered taxi arrived to take us to see the Doctor.

'So,' said the taxi driver, as the rain began falling, 'where would you like to go?'

'*The Doctor Who Experience*, please,' I said, 'and step on it!'

I didn't say 'step on it', actually, but I really wish I had. With all the parking kerfuffle, we were running out of time. Our slot to get into the exhibition was booked for 1.30–2.00 p.m. and it was already approaching the latter.

The driver looked blank. 'Where's that?' he asked. *Brilliant*, I thought: *just what we need*. All those millions of loyal viewers, all the hype, all the buzz, and we find a cab driver (in

Cardiff, where the whole thing began) who doesn't know where the *Doctor Who* exhibition is.

Yet we made it, and, once in there (out of the rain), we had a fine time. If you're a fan, and don't need a parking space, I can recommend it. As for the rest – well, the architecture's stunning, and people were really welcoming. But as for the parking – well, a word to the wise: if you're thinking of heading there, leave the car and take your Tardis.

31 August 2012

In contrast, I end the month by having a ball. Well, playing with a few, anyway. 'Play table tennis again' is on the list for the simple reason that it's something I played a lot when I was in college and still standing. I've never tried to do it from a wheelchair. There's also the familiar grip issue: I don't want to take anyone out via the medium of a flying bat. But, as ever, good old sticky bandage sorts that. I sometimes wonder if I should ask the CMT organization if they'd like me to run a masterclass on sticky tape and its many applications. I like to think my dad would be proud, too. I often think of him and what he taught me when I'm addressing my CMT problems, remembering what he said to me about just getting on with it and concentrating on what you can do, rather than what you can't. Those few words of common sense still resonate for me daily, particularly if I find myself getting frustrated.

And I'm pleased to report that I wasn't half bad. Not a patch on my patient partner, Linda, it must be said, and not quite up to the standard of my college days, obviously, but with a little practice and a plentiful supply of Micropore, who knows? When are the next Olympics, again?

And August doesn't end just on that physical high note, either. There's an unexpected emotional high as well. That evening, relaxing by listening to some music on my iPad, something unexpected happens to me. I'm listening to songs written by the talented evangelical singer/songwriter Graham Kendrick, whose music I used to drum to often, back when I was attending church. It didn't matter that I stopped going; I never stopped listening, because his songs are easy to listen to, just as much as they are to drum to; and though, with only one working vocal cord, I don't sing along too much, in Graham's case I make an exception.

And as I listen, one lyric in particular really speaks to me. 'Is anyone thirsty?' it keeps asking, and I ponder it for a while. What does he mean when he asks that? I begin to think I understand. It certainly makes me start thinking about my own faith – or rather lack of it. It's been absent for a long time now, and up till recently I've been comfortable with that. I've been content. Nothing's been missing in my life. Or has it? I don't know. All I know is that the issue has started to play on my mind lately, and, as a consequence of thinking about it, I am beginning to look at things a little differently. Am I thirsty? Is that it? I think I might be. I don't know where that's going to take me yet, but one thing is clear: I am definitely up for the journey.

SEPTEMBER

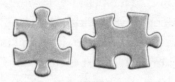

4 September 2012

'He flies like a bird in the sky-eye-eye-eye ...' Yes, you
  probably do have to be a certain age to read that and start
  singing, but it's the first thing that popped into my head, so
  it stays.

My first challenge in a month that I'm hoping will include
plenty of them was to fulfil a lifelong ambition and go up in a
hot air balloon. I'd thought it might be complicated – how
d'you get a wheelchair in a balloon basket? – but, as our pilot
Dave Groombridge explained, this was a special kind of
basket, with a side that folds down to create a ramp. I was also
honoured to be the first passenger for what would be the
balloon's maiden voyage, and had the added pleasure of Lisa
and the children being there to watch us fly.

Not that it was any sort of picnic for them. We took off
from a playing field in Stroud, in Gloucestershire, and, wind
being wind, it was never clear where we'd float. So as my own
giant-sized picnic basket began to float aloft, they had to

hotfoot it back to the car so that they could follow the support crew, who had to do their best to try to follow the balloon …

Up in the sky, however, I was pretty oblivious to the kind of *Wacky Races* scenario being played out on the ground. The Montgolfier brothers knew what they were about, because there is nothing quite like ballooning; there really isn't. The lift-off was so graceful I could hardly sense it. I was looking up at the burner at the time and was staggered to then look down and find we'd been lifted 100 feet up in the air in a matter of seconds.

We eventually attained a height of around 3,000 feet and the view of the Gloucestershire countryside was stunning. I recorded it, too: I had treated myself to my own GoPro camera with this very challenge in mind, a little gift from me to me that I know will keep on giving and which meant, once they had tracked us down, that Lisa and the kids could at least get a sense of just how magical it was up there. Definitely their turn to do it next!

8 September 2012

Number of challenges now complete: 23.

Aren't people kind? When I added 'Go to the Proms' to my list, I was happy to go to any of them. I certainly didn't have the last night in mind; everyone knows tickets for that particular one are like gold dust. But a phone call and an email earlier in the year paid dividends: I was allowed to order tickets for what's normally a sell-out night, and for both me and Lisa, which made it doubly special.

My wife deserves medals for all sorts of things – marrying a mad guy like me, for starters – but this year she deserves a whole trunkful. And not just for the patience she's shown in putting up with my adventures. She also deserves one for enduring the stress I don't doubt my doing them has put her under. It's one thing to be inconvenienced by your husband's frequent absences as he goes off to complete a bunch of crazy challenges, but quite another to have to live with the anxiety that one day he might come home injured or incapacitated. I couldn't have wished for a more supportive wife.

So I decided to treat her as well. Dressed up to the nines (and somewhat boiled, in the warm early-autumn sunshine), first we dined in the Royal Albert Hall's Elgar Restaurant, which was magical. I'm no food critic – except when it comes to crèmes brûlées, obviously – but delicious is delicious in any language. Yes, I should perhaps have taken out a small mortgage to cover the cost of it, but when in Rome and all that. Got to be done. Ditto the delicious champagne cocktails.

The concert itself was fantastic. We were sitting right next to the percussion, yet the acoustics were so good that we weren't deafened; and we could hear every instrument so clearly. The only thing I didn't understand was why the conductor kept on going off stage at the end of every piece, or movement, or whatever they call each bit of music. Comfort break? You can tell I'm not an expert.

But, again, you don't need to be an expert to enjoy things, and when the orchestra played 'Rule Britannia', the sound of thousands of voices singing in unison made the hairs on the back of my neck stand up. Hundreds of Union Jack flags were waved – a sea of red, white and blue. In fact, the woman behind me got a bit carried away with hers and kept smacking me on the head with it.

But I am happy to forgive her. It was *such* a great evening.

10 September 2012

Number of Union Jack waistcoats now in my possession: 1.
Number of occasions I can see when I'm likely to wear it
   again: 0.
Ergo, time to log on to eBay …

There are lots of reasons why I embarked on The 50 List, obviously, but with a new school year under way, my mind today is very much on one reason in particular – the main reason I did it, in fact: my youngest daughter. For Mattie and Amy, there will be all the usual challenges that go with school life – new teachers, new ambitions perhaps, important exams looming – but for Ellie this period will be more challenging than for most, as she's about to transfer to a new school.

It's not going to be full time – she'll still attend her existing primary in the afternoons – but in a week's time she'll start attending a different school in the mornings, Rowan Gate, which is more geared to helping with her additional educational needs in Maths and English. But it's not only about getting extra help with the core subjects. It will, we hope, also prepare her for the next big challenge she's going to be facing: next year she will be attending a specialist secondary school, as I did, and the mornings at Rowan Gate are designed to make that transition easier.

But we have a feeling she's not going to enjoy it.

Today, however, Ellie is all smiles and so are we. That's because, in what I often think is some sort of act of organized insanity, her teachers, plus several brave (or foolhardy) assistants, are taking the whole year group of 60 children on a five-day trip to a local activity centre. There they'll have a chance to try all sorts of physical challenges, including canoe-building, abseiling, climbing and high ropes, as well as various team-building activities.

We know Ellie's nervous about doing them, just as much as she's excited, and as we wave off the coach, so are we. It's the first significant amount of time she'll have spent away from the family, but as the coach sweeps past us, though several of her friends are in tears, to my huge relief I see that Ellie isn't one of them. Perhaps seeing me do The 50 List is already paying dividends ...

11 September 2012

Hopes of arranging my challenge to spend a weekend with a
    Formula 1 team: High.
Fingers currently crossed: The full complement.

Where, on this journey, would I have been without friends? I think that time and again, and as I drive to today's activity – a tour of the Force India Formula 1 team factory – I am thinking it again, because today's trip has been made possible by my friend Graham Raphael. He runs an organization called Motorsport Endeavour, which arranges for injured army personnel to experience motorsport and fast cars, and has kindly let me tag along. And I'm very grateful. This might be the perfect opportunity to meet Force India's marketing person and tell him (or her) about The 50 List and then, if I'm lucky, persuade him to let me complete my challenge.

But in a turnaround reminiscent of the day I had to wave goodbye to my Mustang, it seems my hopeful mood is about to be replaced by something less edifying: cause to reflect on my own limitations.

It's on the dual carriageway that it happens, on the way there. One minute I'm happily driving along in the outside lane, looking forward to my day; the next there's a huge lorry moving across from the inside lane straight in front of me.

I have no idea why he'd do this – he's only travelling at around 50 mph – but I have no time to ponder whys and wherefores. I need to focus all my energies on not ploughing into the back of him, because I'm travelling considerably faster. So I do what anyone else would: I slam my foot down on the brake. Only nothing happens. It's as though I don't even have any brakes, and in a panicky instant I realize that my knee doesn't have the power to press my foot down because it's been worn out by all the stop-starts in heavy traffic earlier.

I try again, pumping my leg in the hope of eking out some last vestige of muscle power. But there's still nothing there – nothing that'll do anything in time, anyway – and as I'm fast approaching the back of the lorry, I have no choice but to swerve out of its way. I have no intention of meeting the barrier to the right, which leaves me with a swerve to the left, and the prospect of hitting whatever it was that caused the lorry to pull out in front of me.

My heart's thumping now, but as I pull out from behind the lorry, I see nothing. The lane ahead is empty, which is a major relief. But it also begs a question: why on *earth* did he pull out on me in the first place?

I think it's that point, more than anything, that shakes me up the most. I might feel I'm in control, but I have no control over others. Though the little Mazda handles brilliantly (its handling might just have been a life-saver), its brakes clearly need more muscle power than I, from time to time at least, have in my leg. And suppose the next time I'm forced to brake so hard turns out to be one of those times, and suppose the road ahead is not clear – what then?

I manage to slow the car eventually, and as I do so, it really hits me that I've been so lucky. And that this is not a situation in which anyone – least of all me – should push their luck. Much as I love my classic sports car, I love being alive a whole lot more. When I arrive at Force India, I decide that as soon as I'm home again, I'm going to start looking for a new car.

13 September 2012

*Random observation: The whole house is eerily quiet, even
    though there are still two teenagers in residence.*
*Random discovery: Ah, finally got it! So that's what it is – the
    permanent background drone of the Disney Channel is
    missing ...*

17 September 2012

Sometimes being right is a good thing, sometimes not. We
were right in anticipating that Ellie would have a great time on
her adventure break: she did. Her highlight was the giant
swing – 'It was 40 FEET TALL, Dad!' – and we were very
impressed to hear she'd even tried abseiling. Not for long,
admittedly, because it was obviously very scary, but she did it;
she tried it – she had a go. So she's come home with a bag
stuffed with dirty washing and a head stuffed with lovely
memories, which is exactly as it should be.

But now it's over, and it's much less of a good thing to
know that our prediction about the new school is already
looking like being true as well.

Ellie's first morning at Rowan Gate does not go well, even
though, ultimately, the school will probably be a good thing
for her and we've chatted to her about why going there will be
the sensible thing to do. Martindale liberated me in so many
ways, both expected and unexpected, and though my transition to Martindale was for different reasons (mine were

mostly physical, whereas Ellie's are educational and social), Lisa and I still feel confident that this will be the case for Ellie with Rowan Gate too. After all, it's run to give children with additional needs help they can't access properly in the mainstream. It only accepts pupils who have SENs (Statements of Educational Need), and the pupils are a mixed bunch, as well. Some have conditions such as cerebral palsy or Down's syndrome, others have Asperger's or behavioural problems; some are profoundly disabled.

This will be a totally new experience for Ellie, but her mainstream school, which has done this with previous year-six pupils, believes it will help her. As we do. Just as I've tried to incorporate dexterity challenges into my list to help Ellie remain positive about her diminishing hand and leg strength without being too obvious about it, so the school thinks a gradual transition to the idea of moving to her special secondary school will be best. For the first time she will meet children who have additional needs, as she does, and we hope she will make friends who – unlike the other pupils at her current primary school – will go on to secondary school with her. The plan is that when she's 11, she will attend Friars School, a specialist high school for pupils with special educational needs. And there's another potential bonus, in terms of Ellie's confidence: attending Rowan Gate will mean that for the first time in her life she will know how it feels to be one of the more able children in a class.

But it's clearly going to be a delicate transition. Ellie does her morning at Rowan Gate; then Lisa takes her back to her regular school for lunch and the afternoon session. And when

Lisa returns from dropping Ellie off I can tell by her expression that it's not gone very well.

'So how was she?' I ask.

Lisa frowns. 'Not very happy. She just doesn't understand why she has to go there.'

I can see why Ellie would think that, to be fair. She doesn't know anyone, she doesn't yet fully accept that she needs to go there, and she hates being separated from her friends.

'Jodie particularly,' Lisa says, sighing. 'She's *really* upset about that.'

As she would be, I think, because Jodie is her best friend. As anyone would be. My poor little girl.

18 September 2012

Not a great start to the day. Ellie does not want to return to her new school for the morning. She didn't enjoy her first day and doesn't understand why we are putting her through this.

We insist she goes, but on her return she's upset. She tells us tearfully that she can't remember anyone's name or find her way around the school. Although Matt, a helper from her mainstream school, has gone with her for support, he's new himself, so it's not even as if he's a familiar face; on top of everything else, she's trying to get to know him.

All of which is hard. It's one thing to cope with such transitions yourself, and looking back to when I was Ellie's age, I think I coped very well. But it's quite another when it's not you but someone you love – so much harder. So very much harder.

I have a challenge booked to do today, as well. Perhaps ironically, it's 'Fly an aerofile kite'. And since wanting Ellie to fly is what's behind the traumas we're currently putting her through, it feels kind of apt that it takes place close to Rowan Gate school; indeed, as Lisa picks her up to take her back to her usual school for lunch, they get to see us as we do it.

And it's enjoyable, both as a distraction from worrying about how Ellie's coping and because it's nothing like trying to fly the kites of my youth, which would knife straight into the ground as soon as they looked at you. An aerofoil kite such as the one I fly can get airborne with even the gentlest of winds. In fact, the problem is more likely to be the opposite one. Wheelchair kite surfing was never on my list of 50 challenges, but after today, I think it might be by default.

19 September 2012

Ellie is on the verge of hysteria this morning. Her new class at Rowan Gate go swimming each Wednesday and Ellie is adamant that she does not want to go swimming with them. Not that she doesn't love swimmming – she does, and always has. It's one of the things I was most anxious to teach her from a young age, because I knew she'd appreciate, as I do, that sense of being on a level playing field with everyone else; how, in the water, she can forget about her legs.

But I understand her reticence about going with her new school, given that she will be among strangers. Since she's had her operation she is very conscious of her scars and her lack of muscle tone, and is anxious about people staring.

Not that Ellie is telling us any of this today; we just know it. She is complaining of feeling ill, but because we already know how much she dreads the thought of having to go swimming, we are fairly sure this is an excuse to try to get out of it. In the end, the only solution is for us both to go into school with her and, after a discussion about the issues around the operation, the teacher agrees that she doesn't have to swim this week.

20 September 2012

Things are really not getting any better. This morning Ellie is complaining of a tummy ache again and saying she's too ill to go to school. It's hard. No one wants to see their child needlessly distressed, but at the same time we need her to become resilient against life's knocks. We keep reassuring her that, in the long term, this will be a positive step, and in the end, albeit with a few tears along the way, we get her there.

She returns home that day, however, in no better a mood, and once again I understand how she feels. This time she's anxious about children whom she doesn't (yet) know coming up and hugging her at playtime; she doesn't want her personal space invaded, which Lisa and I both agree is reasonable. Plus there's the additional issue – and it's one I can empathize with – that if someone comes up and touches her and catches her by surprise, there's a possibility of her losing her balance and falling over.

21 September 2012

Number of challenges completed after today's: 25. Can't believe I am finally halfway through them!

Before I can do today's challenge, I have to prioritize a bigger one. Lisa and I go into school with Ellie again this morning, to speak to her teacher about the unwanted hugging. Which actually turns out to be plain sailing. Her support teacher, Matt, is given anti-hugging responsibilities and, feeling more supported, Ellie trots off to start her day.

Another hurdle jumped, and I'm off to do the business of the day, which will be more plain sailing, I hope, because I'm off to sail a boat. And though, after that pun, it would obviously be altogether far too cheesy to start musing on the metaphorical business of 'setting sail', as I head out onto the water with Roy Child, the chair of Northamptonshire Sailability, I do have a sense of setting sail on an adventure, as I did when I first decided to create my personal must-do list.

I also recall thinking – and even saying, if I remember rightly – that as one door closes (in this case on my job, when I was made redundant) another one usually opens. And how true that's turned out to be. As doors go, this one's been such a big colourful one: a gateway to a wealth of incredible opportunities. But at the same time, with less than three months to go now, I'm tired. Happily tired, yes, but now that I can see the finish line, I want to be there. Like a marathon runner with a mile to go, tasting the end but knees buckling, I want to *be* at the finish line (in first place, naturally), looking back on it all with pride.

22 September 2012

Number of challenges now complete: A stress-relieving 27.
   Well, give or take the odd ongoing challenge, anyway.
   (Other tallies are, of course, available.)

In times of stress it's always good to get physical. There's nothing like taking out your frustrations on a lump of dough. Though challenge (oh, insert your own number, why don't you?) – 'Bake bread on a regular basis' – is nothing like taking out my frustrations on a lump of dough.

In reality (and this is strictly between us and Ellie, obviously) it has turned out to be a bit of a cheat, this bread-making lark. Tradition has it that the best bread is lovingly hand-made, and that in the kneading the baker will find calm and inner peace. Which is great in theory but, much as I applaud those who devote hours to the business of artisan bread-making, I cottoned on quite quickly that there's an easier way to do it: namely, buy a bread-maker, fill it with bread mix and plug it in – leaving the artisan free to pursue other, less knuckle-wearyingly athletic tasks, such as trying to coax a recalcitrant daughter with the world on her shoulders into helping you to finish the 1,000-piece jigsaw that you started back in February and which is – infuriatingly – still nowhere near being finished.

Which sort of achieves the same purpose on the stress-relieving front, for both of us. The bread bakes, the jigsaw inches (albeit slowly) towards completion, and the net result (as well as the kids having home-made bread in their school lunch boxes) is that I am marginally less agitated by the humiliating spectre of letting all those august engineers down. At least two of them built whole *trains*, for goodness' sake. Whereas my claim to fame (Ellie's too) on the bread-making front is having once made a loaf in the bread-maker, only to forget all about its existence. Forget, that is, till a couple of weeks later, when it began making its presence felt …

24 September 2012

Another week, another episode of school refusal. After a weekend when she hasn't felt ill at all, Ellie is again complaining of feeling poorly. We get her to school, just about. Then I spend time on the phone speaking to the special needs co-ordinator about exactly what we are trying to achieve here.

As someone who had to attend a 'special school' myself, I can sympathize with Ellie. Being segregated from long-standing friends and thrown into a totally new situation is horrible, and though schools for children with special needs have come an awfully long way since the 1970s when I attended one, it's no less stressful to be parted from your friends now, even if it is for just half a day.

Although this wasn't instigated by us, Lisa and I do support it. Yes, it's stressful, but we believe that will be vastly outweighed by the positives. Fingers crossed our trust isn't misplaced.

26 September 2012

Oh, dear. And so it goes on ... Today we have more tears about swimming. Nothing for it: we go into school. Again. For all that we support the business of Ellie being there, this is clearly going to be a sticking point. Over something that matters not a jot.

And it's worth it. This time the teacher takes one look at Ellie's tear-stained face and agrees that there will be no swimming at all, ever. This is in contrast to the special needs co-ordinator, who insisted that Ellie could not be allowed to win this battle and 'must' go swimming, as she has to learn that she can't always have her own way.

There's another issue here. One of the key reasons for Ellie going here was so that she could concentrate on Maths and English. She has no need of swimming lessons anyway. She had swimming lessons last year and is a perfectly good swimmer; she goes almost every week already with me, Matt and Amy.

We leave the meeting feeling happier that someone has listened to us. All this talk of battles and the rights or wrongs of Ellie getting her own way, when, actually, it was an unnecessary stress for her. Now it's mended, let's hope things start to get better.

Ellie's not the only thing that's been on my mind these past days. Perhaps it's because I've been reflecting on her current troubles, or perhaps it's the culmination of a process that's been going on for months – I'm not sure. All I know is that I've found myself engaged in a private dialogue with the guy upstairs.

It's been going on a little while now, ever since I listened to those songs a couple of weeks back. I wonder if doing The 50 List has been a catalyst for moving me towards whatever plan he has mapped out for me. I don't know, but what I do know is that lately I've been realizing that all the time my faith's been absent, God hasn't gone anywhere. It's not that there is no God; it's just that I had lost my faith. And for a simple reason: that my prayers weren't being answered. But was he ignoring me? No. I don't think that any more. I'm beginning to understand that I had been praying for the wrong things. I should have been asking God to help me through the tough times; to help keep me strong, and to guide me.

Being a lay pastoral minister, Lisa's always wanted me to return to the church, but as I made clear when we chatted about it recently, if I ever came back to the church, it wouldn't be for my wife – it would be for me. And it's a work in progress; I need to be sure that I'm returning for the right reasons. But here I am, praying for strength and guidance, to help us through Ellie's current travails. It feels right. It feels not so much that I've found a missing link but as if I've stumbled upon one I didn't even know I'd lost. And that feels pretty good in itself.

All of the above said, though, I'll never be the model churchgoer. I'm not a fan of pomp and ceremony, and sometimes I can be a little irreverent. I also have a short attention span, when it comes to sermons. I have even walked out of a service before now, halfway through a sermon, simply because I got very bored. Don't get me wrong: they aren't all like that. Just some of them …

I also prefer to keep my relationship with God between Him and me. I'm not one to go Bible bashing or shoving scripture down people's throats. I hate it when people try that with me and I'm not one to hold back my feelings when they do try to ram it down my throat when I'm not expecting it. If someone asks me about my faith, however – well, of course, that's different. Then I'll tell them. Of course I will. Gladly.

And I don't know what it is about being a wheelchair user, but as I'm sure other wheelchair users will testify, it tends to attract the patters and the benders – and particularly when I go to church. I don't like to sound grumpy, but as I imagine any normal person would, I hate being approached and patted on my shoulder by people I don't know. I know why they do it: it's because I'm at a suitable height. I don't think they'd do it if I were standing up. I also dislike people coming up to me when I'm in church and bending down in front of me in a patronizing manner, as if I were a child in a pushchair. Fortunately there aren't too many of those.

Perhaps it's just as well, because, faced with a patter or bender, I'm not normally one to hold my tongue: I dive right on in and tell them. Perhaps I need to be a little more tolerant about such things when I hit 50. On the other hand … Nah. Perhaps not!

OCTOBER

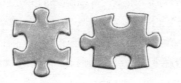

18 October 2012

Time to take a look at progress on the jigsaw. Hmm. What to say? No, it's obviously not done yet. That said, there seems to be a blue train emerging on the left. Thought it was going to be late but, actually, it seems to be coming in on time. In other areas, I'd obviously be happier if I could just find Isambard Kingdom Brunel's midriff, but it is nowhere to be found. BERRY!

Looking down at my steam engines, it occurs to me that although I'm not finished yet, I've made progress on several of the other 'ongoing' fronts, not all of them requiring long periods hunched over a coffee table looking for body parts of famous engineers.

One of the less physical challenges I set myself was 'Make my business work'. This has been both as a necessity (that pesky mortgage) and to set an example to my children that, whether you work for yourself or someone else, it's all down to you; that the key is to take pride in everything you do and

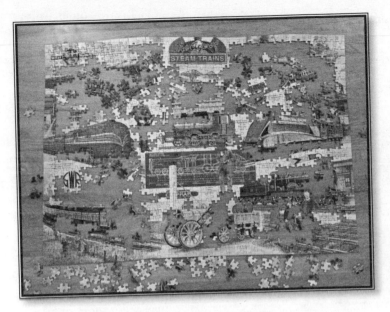

The puzzle that haunts me every time I pass it. It WILL be finished!

always do the very best you can. For Amy, I had a chance to do some hands-on stuff as well. When her school had a 'go to work with Dad' day back in the spring, she spent hers learning how I design some of my websites, and also helped create a business logo. So far, the challenge has been a success. Though completing the list has meant having to hold off on taking on major projects, we're now into October – a whole year since I left my last position – and I can honestly say my fledgling business is working and it is growing.

Though I am not. And as one of my other ongoing challenges was 'Lose weight', this is excellent news. True, I've not lost much weight (I'm not even that far into single figures) but I am eating more thoughtfully, and as a consequence more healthily.

I also feel I can award myself a tick for two further ongoing challenges: 'Cover FIA drag-racing events in Europe for our online magazine' and 'Donate funds raised through The 50 List to the CMT organization'. With the former, it might not have been to the extent that I'd have liked (running an online magazine is a time-consuming and costly business, and, for the moment, at least, we've had to put it on hold), but I covered the first round of the European Championships, at least. As for CMT, well, that's very much a work in progress. I've already raised £1,000 for them, but I'm not stopping there. I've aimed high – my target is £5,000 – but I have absolutely no doubt that I'll get there. I have to: they badly need money to survive. And survive they must, as they do such an exceptional job in making people aware of the condition, providing support and helping fund research.

25 October 2012

Phew. Number of bits of wood successfully turned: 3 – 2 by me. Number of digits still intact: The full 9. Oh, hang on ...

Is there something about people who work with wood, I wonder? Some indefinable trait they all share? I have no idea, but whatever it is, it's worth having, because woodworkers always seem to be at peace with themselves and with the world, and uncommonly nice.

I loved woodwork classes at Martindale; loved everything about them. I loved the woodworking workshop, perhaps because it didn't feel like school. A single-storey prefab of the kind that was common in the 1960s and 1970s, it sat apart from the main buildings and had far-reaching views – one of the adjacent primary school, and the other of our own school's extensive playing fields. I loved the smell: because of all the wood kept in the storeroom, it always smelled like a forest, with pleasing occasional top notes of wood glue. I loved the layout – the twin rows of three heavy wooden benches, each with its own vice and neat set of tools, just waiting for you to come along and play with them. I loved the sense of anticipation, the idea that you could take a block of wood and, using just your hands and the tools you had in front of you, create something both beautiful and useful.

But mostly, I really liked our woodwork teacher. A genial chap in his late sixties (with obviously no thought of retirement), he was like a friendly uncle, always smiling and in a freshly pressed white coat, and with two pencils, always, in his top pocket. He lived to teach, and to pass on his passion for working with wood, telling us endless stories as we worked about various students past, in the hope of inspiring us to make woodworking our careers.

Some of his stories were far-fetched, though. I remember one about a young man he had in his class for an afternoon, and who was floundering in life, unable to find work.

'So I taught him to change a window frame,' he told us. 'In that single afternoon. And it turned out to be the making of the lad. The very next day he went out and changed window frames for several people, and went on to make a very good living.'

None of us quite believed that (we had the evidence of our own efforts to remind us that woodwork wasn't that easy), but it didn't seem to matter. He used the stories like a tool – perhaps a slightly blunt chisel, but they did their job, as we always came out inspired.

The thing I really hankered after was using the lathe, the piece of machinery – and we had several big pieces in our classroom – that seemed the king among woodworking tools. And when my turn came (I made a light stand, shortly before leaving school for college) it was every bit as thrilling and manly to use as I'd imagined. The light stand itself was possibly less thrilling, it must be admitted, but it stayed at my mum's right up until she passed away, by which time it had been painted some lurid shade of blue or green by one of my brothers. It then made its way, via a car boot sale, to a new home, where I like to think it's still doing sterling service.

*   *   *

Woodworking, then, was always a natural fit for me, because I knew it would bring back many happy memories. So I was thrilled that my various 50 List enquiries bore fruit, in the form of an email from a guy called Mike Donovan, the vice chairman of the Association of Wood Turners of Great Britain. As well as having a cracking title, Mike was both generous and super-talented, and graciously allowed me to go to his home and use his lathe, and in doing so create some beautiful things.

I made two pieces. The first was a chess piece – a pawn – and the second, with Mike's help as my hands were tiring, a vase, made from a piece of yew. The hard part was the sanding, which you do while the lathe is turning, holding the sandpaper while the wood spins around. Or, in my case, half the time not holding: with my lack of grip, it kept wanting to leave my hands and go for a spin itself around the workroom.

Finally, a joint effort, made to my design by Mike: a beautiful Brazilian rosewood bowl, with a penny coin inlaid in the base – from 1962, the year I was born.

But wouldn't you know it? Everyone's a critic.

'You won't get far playing chess with just one piece,' Lisa quipped, when I proudly unveiled my pawn. 'Are you going back to make the other 15?'

Oh well, I thought, *at least they'll be impressed by the vase.* Which they were, kind of, though there was a distinct lack of gush. That's the thing with families: they keep your feet on the ground at all times.

And so to the bowl.

'Look,' I said to Ellie. 'See that coin there in the bottom? That was minted the same year I was born.'

She peered in to look. 'Yes, but what's the point of it?' she wanted to know. 'Soon as you pour in your cornflakes, you won't be able to see it, will you?'

27 October 2012

Number of challenges now completed including this one: 34.
    Oh, yeah. Cracking through them now at the speed of light.
    Well, sort of.
Puzzle watch: Day 300 and … Oh, I've lost count now. All I
    know is that there's quite a bit of red train still to complete.
    And that I hate all red trains ever built. Ever.
However, in other news: Finally, we zorb!

Of all the things I'd like to teach my kids, Ellie in particular, the most important is that you don't know if you're going to like something, or be good at something, or hate it with a passion, till you've actually gone and tried it for yourself.

There's only so much you can get from watching other people doing something, after all. And in some cases, watching someone else doing something can give you the wrong impression, as what something looks like isn't necessarily what it *feels* like.

And so to zorbing, one of my most eagerly anticipated challenges, and which, on this bright if not particularly breezy autumnal Saturday, we are about to do.

I say 'we', but Ellie's not actually with us this morning; she's at home with Lisa. She's still too young and small to have a go at zorbing. Assuming she even wants to.

'But do you think you'd like try it?' I asked her when I scheduled it on my calendar. 'You know, when you're old enough to have a go at it yourself?'

She thought for all of two seconds. It might even have been less. Then shook her head.

'No,' she said. 'No, I definitely wouldn't.'

'Any particular reason?' I asked her. Ellie always has a reason. She might be quiet but she thinks about things.

It turned out that in this case it was actually reasons, plural. 'Because I don't like going upside down,' she said. 'Because I don't like rolling really fast. And because I get car sick, so I expect I would be roll sick.'

So that was clear, then. And logical. Also I have to hand it to her: my Ellie definitely knows her own mind.

And perhaps, as it turns out, I should have known better too. That's something I begin thinking almost as soon as we arrive in Croydon and find that my satnav has directed us to a forest. Now, you can say what you like about Croydon, and I know a lot of people do, but I have no axe to grind in that respect. It's just that I was expecting something a little more – how can I put it? – *organized* than what we're currently faced with. A building at least, perhaps with the words 'Come zorbing!' emblazoned across it. At the very least some sign of human life.

'You sure we're in the right place, Dad?' Mattie says as we park in what seems to be the designated area. Looking around, I have my doubts. But then Amy spots a procession of tiny signs, affixed to trees, which apparently point the way to where the zorbing happens, which, of necessity, must be at the top of a hill. Which we almost are, so we clamber out – me, in my wheelchair, Matt and his friend Sam, who's joining us, and Amy – and follow the path in the direction the arrows seem to be pointing. I say 'path'; it's not so much a path as a twig-strewn green carpet – literally, a green carpet, half buried under piles of rotting leaves, much infiltrated by mud, and marked out at either side by bits of wood. It's such a mess that I only find out later that it's a carpet, on enquiring why they don't just lay some tarmac. They can't. They're not allowed to lay a proper path here, as it's a place of nature, which is presumably why at its end the only man-made structure is a small wooden kiosk, close to the top of a vertiginous incline.

It's bitterly cold today, and we get colder as we stand and book in. As we do so we see zorbing balls rolling down the hill. At this point it still looks exciting to all of us. Next up is to get on and do it. To ride in a zorb ball you have to be strapped in, obviously, and you are harnessed on your back, with someone else on the opposite side, both of you lying on your backs with your knees bent. Affixed as you are at both upper body and ankles, it seems comfortable and sturdy enough. I'm even looking forward to the experience a little – not least to the photos we'll be able to look at afterwards, as we have brought the GoPro camera that I treated myself to in the summer, and I've affixed it to Amy's head.

All that done, Amy and I are ready for the off (Matt and Sam will be going down after us) and I finally feel just a little bit nervous. But nervous in a good way? That's how it usually happens. Will it happen that way now? We shall see.

And I do see. So, then, how to describe zorbing? Well, unless you've been a jumper in a tumble dryer, it's a little tricky. But if you are of an imaginative bent, I'm sure you can improvise. Happily, unlike a jumper, I'm mostly fixed in position, though not completely: my chest and my feet are fairly stable, but the rest of me, from waist to knee, is attached to nothing very much as we flip and flop our way, father and daughter, down that tree-lined Croydon hill, so had we been jumpers, we would have come out very dry ones.

As well as speed, there is excitement. A slightly nervous excitement, it must be said, as it stems from the fact that the camera unclips from Amy's forehead almost as soon as we start descending. It's still held by its strap, but it lends a real frisson to the experience to know that it might at any point become completely detached from her and spend its own journey down repeatedly hitting the pair of us in or on any body part fate chooses.

And the thrills don't end at the bottom of the hill. We roll to a stop, Amy laughing her head off – yup, she loved it – but we've stopped in such a way that I'm now suspended in the worst possible position, hanging so that all my bodyweight is pulling down on my legs. With my condition I cannot kneel, so the pain is excruciating, and it's all I can do not to cry out in agony. But I manage to ask the young guy now in charge of de-zorbing us if he can roll us so that I'm lying on my back.

That done, my darling daughter is now hanging there above me, still giggling. Which makes me realize that there *is* such a thing as having too much fun.

'Shall I undo my straps, Dad?' she quips, clearly oblivious to my suffering.

'No!' I scream. And it *is* a scream. 'You'll land on top of me!'

'How was that?' asks the chirpy young man charged with freeing me from this extra torture. Which elicits another small scream, but I still manage to be polite.

'Well,' I say diplomatically, 'let's just say I won't be doing it again in a hurry. Now get me out of here, please.'

Which, mercifully, he does. And I'm not even a celebrity.

So, zorbing. Why did I do it? Well, as I tell Ellie afterwards, I did it because it was something I'd never done before, and the only way I was going to find out if I liked it was to try it.

'So would you do it again?' she asks, as we sit and do some work on the jigsaw together.

'Oh, yes,' I tell her. 'Just not in this lifetime.'

NOVEMBER

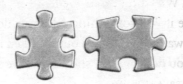

1 November 2012

Number of challenges to squeeze in between now and the end
of the month: 5.
Number of quarts that can reasonably be fitted into a pint pot:
Erm ...
OK, let's just say too many, shall we? No time for dithering
around here, thinking up things to say about stuff. I have a
deadline to meet, remember?

So. First up, today we all went to the West End of London to
see a show. I was keen to include something of this kind, not
only because of the fun aspect – though, heck, why wouldn't
anyone want to do that? – but also because it would, I hoped,
provide evidence for Ellie that having added complications
when getting around (in a city like London, particularly)
should never preclude her from doing anything she wants to
do, even if it might occasionally preclude her from making the
odd train. That certainly happened to me a couple of times,
back in the day. Crawling up and down the steps at stations is

not to be recommended as a pastime generally, so it's good to see how much better London's transport infrastructure is these days.

So off we all went, to see *Shrek the Musical*. No, it wasn't my first choice – I really wanted to go and see *Stomp*. Or, if that was fully booked, perhaps *War Horse* – I fancied that. Or, at a pinch, *Jersey Boys*. But, no, I know my place; I was overruled and outnumbered. So *Shrek the Musical* it was. And it was brilliant.

8 November 2012

Getting there ... 36 down, 5 still ongoing. Which means we're into single figures now – wahey!

Today I piloted a narrow boat, which was great fun. And the key thing to know here is that back in the mid-1980s or thereabouts, I actually turned down tickets to see David Bowie at the National Bowl in Milton Keynes in order to do just such a thing. I know; I can't quite believe I did that now, either. But actually it was a brilliant weekend. It was supposed to be for 'training', and related to my part-time activities as a youth worker. A bunch of young guys, a boat (name of *Pisces*) and the whole Grand Union Canal on which to play: I don't remember a single thing we did that could be called 'training', only much eating, much drinking and a great deal of fun. Perhaps more fun, looking back, than I'd have had being squished alongside several thousand sweaty people watching a pin-sized David Bowie from a great distance ...

The plan today was for me to have a go at steering exactly the same boat, courtesy of a friend of mine, Simon Cox. When I told him about the challenge and mentioned that I'd once steered a narrow boat called *Pisces*, he laughed out loud.

'I can help you with that!' he assured me. 'Nigel, you know what? This was meant to be.'

Turns out that Simon's aunt, Brenda Hale, works at the Hillingdon Narrowboats Association and looks after all the boats there (which still include *Pisces*), maintaining them and preparing them to go out. It took a few phone calls but Simon was as good as his word, and as a result today I made the trip down to reacquaint myself.

For those of you who enjoy the odd nautical statistic, *Pisces* is 72 feet long and weighs 20 tons. Unfortunately, when we got to the boatyard to take her out, I soon realized that, contrary to the days when I wasn't accessorized by a wheelchair, I could no longer fit in the space at the back. So, instead, I took out *Pisces*'s sister boat *Star*, which had enough space for both me and my trusty wheelchair.

So *Star* was the star of this particular challenge, though it was *Pisces*, ironically, that was on my mind as I left. That was because one of my remaining challenges is 'Catch a big sea fish' – a challenge that's proving a little difficult to complete. Had I thought more, I could have brought a fishing rod ...

10 November 2012

Number of challenges still remaining: 13 – including those in
that 'ongoing' category.
Number of light bulbs used in the Blackpool illuminations
(when they're lit, that is): 400,000. There's a humorous
ironic correlation in there somewhere, I'm sure. Just can't
shed light on it right now. Sorry!

Water. Stuff of life. Where would we be without it? And on a
more personal level, where would The 50 List be? Without
water I'd have been unable to do several of my challenges. The
one two days back, for instance. Plus the jet-skiing. Plus the
scuba diving. In fact, thinking about it, a large number of the
challenges have required water in some shape or form.

Today, though, for a trip to Blackpool I have no need of
water. Nor does Lisa, nor Ellie. Nor does anyone in Blackpool,
frankly, bar the big stuff that sits just off the beach. Yet by
some random meteorological blip (no, Nigel, don't be silly
– this is the North of England in November) we have an
embarras de richesses of the bloody stuff.

It's just the three of us who've travelled up here to complete
today's challenge, which is to visit the famous tower, if only
because, as I think Sir Edmund Hillary said of something else,
it's there. Mattie and Amy are absent because they have both
gone off on a church youth group weekend away. With any
luck, they'll be drier than we are. They'd certainly be hard
pushed to be any wetter. We're only half an hour into our visit
when the heavens open up a hole that must be the size of

Greater Manchester, and the rain starts coming down in quantities that beggar belief.

Still, the tower is impressive in the flesh, even if the top is covered in tarpaulin, and I'm not really disappointed that whatever it is they're doing means we probably wouldn't have been able to go up there. I'm equally pleased that with the rain lashing down so enthusiastically, we're forced to decamp to a fish and chip shop – Harry Ramsden's, no less – instead of being wind-driven down the length of the soaking prom.

Our meal finished, the weather decides to be kind – particularly to Ellie – and gives us a respite long enough for us to make our way to the pier to spend an hour playing games and having fun. But having too much fun is obviously something the Blackpool weather frowns on, as no sooner are we there than it starts raining again, and continues to do so till we get in the car and leave.

And – sorry Blackpool, it's nothing personal – we are happy to. Not just because of the rain but because, sadly, this hasn't been the Blackpool I'd hoped to find. It isn't the bitter cold either; it is just the whole atmosphere. As we drive back to the hotel where we are going to spend the night, what we mostly see are not the illuminations (there are none, bar those required to alert low-flying aircraft) but the numbers of police and drunken youngsters in the town. So, overall, not the brightest or the best of all my challenges. Bit of a damp squib, in fact. Fish and chips were good, though!

15 November 2012

Challenge 38 – go bungee jumping ...

... though the bottom line is: I'm not jumping after all. Well, not intentionally, anyway. Because though I'm now going to be skiing instead, my middle name is not 'The Eagle'. I'm not insane. I'm just going to try the regular downward kind.

I had every intention of doing a bungee jump, but there were a few factors that made me decide that I should try something else. First, this was one activity Lisa really didn't want me to do. She was worried, quite reasonably, that I would do myself some injury. Second, my plan had been to find a bungee jump set-up where I would be in a full body harness rather than just wearing straps around my legs, and it would also have had to be above water and somewhere where I wouldn't need to climb up – all of which were beginning to make it something of a big ask.

Finally, in the back of my mind there is a small nagging directive that goes by the name of an instinct for self-preservation. Much as I'd like Ellie, Matt and Amy to believe anything is possible, there is a limit, and, all things considered, perhaps 'Nigel Holland bungee jumping' goes a teeny bit beyond it.

So skiing it is. And that suits me just fine. I have booked a lesson with Disability Snowsport UK, based at Xscape in Milton Keynes, where there's an indoor snow slope that even has real snow, plus all the paraphernalia to allow a wheelchair user to ski. It also has (if Sam Colby, who looks after me, is anything to go by) instructors who have the patience of saints. And it is great fun. Within no time I am not only rocking but also rolling – in this case, in a generally downward direction (which is desirable) – and feeling that familiar buzz of speed. Yes, I take a tumble a couple of times, but then what skier doesn't? I do OK – by all accounts very well for my first lesson. This is definitely one for all the kids to try.

21 November 2012

Drat. After all my high hopes of ticking off my Formula 1 challenge, I got an email this morning from Force India. Seems that, on this occasion anyway, they can't help me. Which is a great blow, both from the point of view of The 50 List, obviously, but also personally: it was one I really wanted to do.

But never say die. It may yet happen. And it wasn't for lack of trying, which is what the list is all about. Hey ho. Onwards and, well, onwards …

28 November 2012

*An Englishman, an Irishman and a Scotsman walked into a
    bar …*
*… Because the Welshman was still trying to park his car for
    less than a king's ransom in Cardiff. Boom boom!*

I was really looking forward to visiting my final capital city, not least because it meant I could take another flight. I love flying. And, as of now, I also love Belfast. It's absolutely true what they say about Irish hospitality.

I've been lucky with this challenge, too, because I went with my friend Simon Cox, and because of his connections there with Belfast members of Business Networking International (BNI) we received a level of hospitality that we really hadn't expected. Julie Gray, from BNI, was at Belfast City airport to pick us up, which was so helpful, as I'm not too sure what the taxis are like with wheelchairs. From there Julie had arranged with Thomas Fegan, the centre director at Eddie Irvine Sports, for Simon and me to have a go at some go-kart racing.

It had been some years since I'd got behind the wheel of a go-kart but I was willing to give it a bash. I tried a go-kart with hand controls first, but I couldn't get a very good grip; so in the end, sticky bandage being a health-and-safety no-no in this situation, I decided to use a standard go-kart. I had a little more luck with that but didn't feel totally comfortable with the brake pedal, so, given that the 'bash' part might feature rather more than originally intended, I bowed out and left Simon to it.

We got a chance to have a go on some racing simulators, though, and I'm pleased to report that, despite crashing my car and turning it over, I beat Simon. Result! Mind you, thinking about it, coming seventh and eighth out of eight racers is not a lot to write about really. So perhaps I won't.

In the afternoon Julie very kindly gave us a tour of some of Belfast's past trouble spots. Having seen so much of them on television over the years, it was fascinating to see them for real and put them in context. I was very impressed with the murals painted on the sides of buildings and walls. They depict the struggles that went on for years, and are a powerful visual reminder that such struggles should never happen again.

Finally – and unexpectedly – Belfast gave me a perfect opportunity to well and truly nail another challenge: 'Give a talk as a guest speaker'. Actually, though, I'd already ticked this particular box. I've agreed to give a talk to the CMT organization next year, and on a smaller but no less meaningful scale, I recently talked to the local church youth group, called 3:16. I could have talked about me, and The 50 List, which would have been easy, obviously, but I thought it would be nice to give them something more general to chew on. So I used the opportunity to talk to the group about disability, and included my favourite soapbox subject: the difference between being disabled and having a disability.

Belfast was slightly different. I was offered the chance to speak to members of the BNI – at 6.30 in the morning, no less! The format is (and was) that you have 60 seconds to deliver a presentation in which you convey what your business or organization is all about. I spoke about The 50 List, and am proud to report that my talk was unplanned, unscripted and completely off the cuff. So I declare that particular challenge a *big* tick: go me! No, I'm not quite at the stage where I'll be joining the after-dinner speakers' network, but what a confidence boost! Thank you, Belfast!

DECEMBER

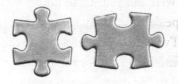

2 December 2012

Number of pieces in place in the 1,000-piece jigsaw: 999.
  Done.

They'll be dancing in the streets of Wellingborough tonight, I'm sure, because – ta da! – the jigsaw is finally finished. Yes, there's a piece missing, but that's fine. Just as, historically, the weavers of Persian rugs felt culturally obliged to stitch in a single mistake as a mark of respect to God, so I am prepared to accept that in any jigsaw-based endeavour, a missing piece is probably appropriate, as evidence of the rigours of the journey travelled.

Plus, it's probably in the dog, so that's the end of it. Score at full time: Nigel and Ellie 1, puzzle 0!

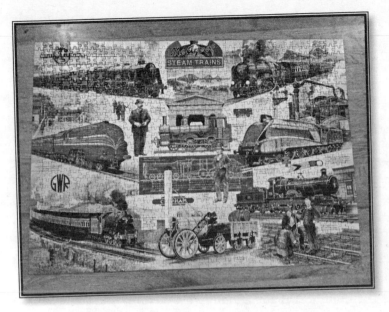

Completed! OK, apart from one piece that was eaten by the dog.

7 December 2012

Challenge on the list: 'Swim 100 lengths of the local pool.'
Challenge in reality: 'Hand-cycle 5 miles uphill.'

I'm not a quitter, me; never was and never will be. So, as with substituting another challenge for the bungee jumping challenge last month, I was somewhat reluctant to swap this one. But sometimes in life you have to take off your superhero overpants and replace them with your sensible hat. The truth is that, with the spell in hospital in the spring, swimming that far in my local pool would be madness. There's also the not-so-small matter of my shoulder. While I passionately believe that anything is possible, that's with the caveat that the thing is not beyond a person's physical limitations. And one of my physical limitations is that I have the kind of dodgy shoulders that require a lot of care and attention.

This is nothing to do with my CMT. Much as I'd like to live in a world where if you get one thing you're automatically exempt from getting another, I have the same cronky shoulders from which thousands of others suffer, more's the pity. I had to have surgery on my right one in 2008 which, as well as meaning that I wore out the carpet by wheeling round in circles for several months, put me physically in a disadvantaged state. And since humans are symmetrical, the left appears to be going the same way.

But there is a relationship between my shoulders and my CMT, in that, being a wheelchair user, I need my shoulders and general arm strength more than most people do, so I have to be realistic and take care. I'm not fit enough to swim 100 lengths, in any case, and even if I were, the cold water in the local swimming pool would give me cramp before too long, and my muscles don't deal well with cramp.

So, reluctantly, I swapped this particular challenge for one that didn't involve me getting wet but would test my stamina instead. I decided that I would try to hand-cycle 5 miles uphill, using the hand-cycle machine at the gym. Not that I let myself off lightly: I set the resistance of the machine high so that I would have to work pretty hard. It took me 30 minutes to cover the 5 miles and I don't think I could have done any more. I kept up a strong pace and only stopped twice – and then only to have more strapping put on my hands, to ensure I could keep a good grip on the handles.

So what am I doing now, at the end of what was still a gruelling challenge, worrying that people might see it as a cop-out? It's not that I need to justify myself, is it? After all, it's not as if I haven't already proved I'm not a quitter. It's not as if I haven't already done a half marathon, is it?

I probably need to stop it, as I know Lisa will tell me, because, actually, what an incredible year it's been! And I'm so excited that it's almost over, not because I've wanted it to finish but because of the way it makes me feel to look back and see what I've achieved. I feel as though I've just won the longest ever marathon in history. Which makes me want to jump up and down, shouting, 'I won! I won!'

It also puts me in a reflective frame of mind. What does it mean to me, this year of madness? Well, one thing's clear: it's really made me focus more on my family. The very idea of it – to show Ellie that anything is possible – has been such a journey. And not just for me and Ellie but for Matthew and Amy, too. I feel I've been able to show all of them what exciting lives they have ahead of them; that the three of them are just so lucky to be alive; and that life is one great big opportunity, waiting to be grabbed.

9 December 2012

My birthday!

OK. As is customary on such occasions, time for a little stock-taking. It's my birthday and I am now 50 years old, but still I refuse to grow up. Looking back, while I lie here waiting for Lisa to bring me my birthday cup of tea in bed, I go through all the crazy things that I have done this year.

Some of them felt easy and natural, and not very challenging at all, and they were such fun: making a crème brûlée, learning to make proper soup. In contrast, some were really 'out there' as challenges go for me: managing to ride a Jet Ski, having a go at indoor skydiving, skiing down a snowy slope, reaching 160 mph in about eight seconds and scuba diving in sunny Italy. There have been painful times, too – the most memorable of them being when my knees got bent backwards when I was zorbing, almost causing me to scream in agony. There is a video file of this moment but I have had to consign it to the 'DO NOT USE' folder because every time I see it it's as if the pain returns.

There's also been the quiet joy of some of the more long-term challenges. Passing on my knowledge of website design to Ian, and to Amy on her 'go to work with Dad' day, involved the pure satisfaction of exactly that: passing on a skill. I've also loved curating my very own photo exhibition, to be shown at the Castle Theatre, Wellingborough. No, I'm not the best photographer ever, but I'm not half bad either, and having the skill to capture that moment when a car or bike is travelling close to 300 mph is something that makes me very proud.

I also feel proud that I've finally gone and done it: I've written a proper comedy sketch. Just sneaked it in, close to the wire (you'll find it at the back of this book), and I am full of joy and pride as a result. There is nothing quite like making people laugh, is there?

10 December 2012

Number of years old: 50 and 1/365th.
Number of challenges completed: 46.
Number of challenges that will be completed eventually, if I
*   have anything to do with it: 4.*

Sometimes in life you have to be pragmatic. After all, not everything is under your control (more of which later). Not that I've given up on my four remaining challenges. I still have high hopes of spending a weekend with a Formula 1 team, meeting John Cleese, catching a big sea fish and getting one of my photos printed in a national newspaper. But they're for next year. For this year, I'm done. Done and proud as well. And after the visit to the distillery, the travails in Cardiff, the skiing and the zorbing (note to self, in case of memory loss: *particularly* the zorbing), I don't feel a day over – let me see, now – 97.

And there's obviously the small matter of my 50th birthday bash, as well, which we held last night because it was a

Saturday. It turned out to be something of a double celebration. Whereas I began the year thinking I'd have a party just to celebrate my 50th, I soon realized that, what with everyone pitching in to help me so much with it, the party should celebrate the completion of The 50 List as well. Which meant that by the time we got to it, it had grown fairly radically, to include everyone who needed a proper thank you.

We didn't have it at home, as there wouldn't have been the space. Instead we held it at the Aviator Hotel in Sywell, partly because of the beautiful Art Deco architecture but mainly because it's only ten minutes' drive from where we live. The entertainment was easy. I booked the Lincoln Noel Trio, a jazz band I'd heard play at a local pub back in the spring. They impressed me so much that I booked them there and then.

And what a turnout! Both of my brothers and sisters-in-law came, plus my brother Mark's son, Richard, and it felt that almost all those nearest and dearest to me were there. And I had the best surprise ever when my sister Nicola showed up. Having told me she had too much on to be able to make the trip back to the UK, she'd secretly travelled over specially, all the way from the United States, and between them, all my siblings had managed not to divulge the secret. Seeing her really did leave me lost for words. And then I had too many: how was she? How had her journey been? What time had she left? How long could she stay? It might sound sentimental but seeing Nicola meant the world to me. I was so shocked that I was actually reduced to tears.

So here I am, a day older, a 50-year-old, suddenly. Which is certainly something to try to get my head around; that and the fact that I feel exactly the same as I did at 49 – energetic, up for it, ready for the next challenge ... And I have a new challenge to think about, because our friends the Webb family gave me a voucher to climb over the O2 arena in London – and not just me, either: it includes Lisa, Mattie, Amy and Ellie as well. 'Don't worry – it's wheelchair friendly!' Richard quipped. 'I checked!' At first I thought it must be a wind-up, but apparently it's not. So that's it. Bring it on!

But my most abiding memory of my 50th birthday party takes me back to that day, 15 long months ago, when I asked my youngest daughter to see if she could suggest anything for my 50 List.

I should have expected there to be something going on, of course, because – well, because she's my daughter. And as she's my daughter, and is therefore at least a bit like me, I suppose I would have been surprised if she hadn't had a little something up her sleeve. But when Lisa confirmed that Ellie did have a surprise for me, I genuinely didn't have a clue what to expect. Bit of a wild one, my little girl, even though she looks as if butter wouldn't melt.

It's been interesting to reflect on what this crazy year might have meant to her. I know how I feel: truly blessed. Overwhelmed by all the support I've had; overwhelmed, looking back, by the lifetime of support I've had. I've also had it reconfirmed to me how brilliant my family and friends are. As for Ellie, well, people have asked me precisely that about her: they've wondered if I could tell what effect it was having on her, seeing some of the challenges I've risen to these past months. After all, that's what this journey has mostly been about.

I've sat and pondered and the truth is that it hasn't really had any effect. Not yet. As I say, she's my daughter, and she's grown up seeing me do all sorts of wild and crazy things. She's certainly already a veteran of the drag-racing scene. It'll be later, I think, that it really sinks in for her, when she looks back – perhaps when facing some challenge of her own – and has that confidence that comes from thinking: *Well, if Dad can do it, I can* ... That's what I hope. What I hope for all three of them.

Right then at the party, though, she was just looking impish. And as I glanced at Lisa, Mattie and Amy, and looked around at all my friends and family, I twigged that it was a joke that everyone seemed to be in on. Everyone, that is, except me. As Ellie bore down on me, her beautifully wrapped gift in her hands, my first thought was that it might be something to do with that wretched jigsaw. A scale model of the *Rocket*, perhaps, or a short history of steam trains. The collected musings, perhaps, of Isambard Kingdom Brunel.

I took the package and began opening it. 'So what's this?' I asked her. 'Please don't tell me it's another jigsaw.'

'You mean you don't *know*?' Ellie replied, smiling ever so sweetly. 'Dad, it's your pink hair dye, of course.'

EPILOGUE

It's probably common knowledge that one of the first laws of parenting is that you should never make a promise you can't keep. If there's any doubt, then don't make the promise in the first place. It's hardly rocket science, is it? And that goes for the good things – the new bicycles, the attendance at sports days, the bedtime stories – as well as the bad (never ground a child in haste – it's odds on you'll regret it).

So when I made Ellie that promise, way back at the start of The 50 List, it was in the certain knowledge that, should she still want me to, I'd have to come good on one challenge in particular. And as she did, that's what I did: I dyed my hair pink. For all that I looked ridiculous, I was glad to do it. Not only because it made her laugh (wonderful though the sound of a daughter's laughter is to any father, obviously), but because it might have taught her a lesson that's equally as important as believing that if you try you can achieve anything: that your word is one of the most powerful things you possess.

But dying my hair pink wasn't challenge number 50; it never had been. It had only been on my reserve list (and then grudgingly), as the eagle-eyed among you might have noticed. Which means the list of challenges still falls one short, at 49.

So how about that 50th challenge? The one not yet accounted for? Did I rub it out? Dispense with it? Quietly forget to mention it? Quite the contrary, even though there's been many times when I've felt like it, because – pink hair adventures aside – in some ways it was the most difficult challenge of the lot. It was certainly the most time-consuming – even more so than that wretched jigsaw. And when I reached the end of it (which was considerably less time ago than you might imagine) I remember thinking, with a great deal of conviction, that it was the challenge that demanded the most of me emotionally; the one that was so much harder than I'd ever anticipated.

In fact, it drained me and elated me in roughly equal measure, which I'm told is normal. I know I certainly won't forget it; I can't. It won't let me.

So what is it, this thing that will always remind me of The 50 List? Of this once-in-a-lifetime experience I've just lived?

Yep, you got it. You're holding it in your hands.

THE 50 LIST

Do an indoor skydive
Go powerboating
Take a 4x4 off road
Play the drums
Teach someone to balance on two wheels in a
    wheelchair
Take part in a half marathon
Make a crème brûlée
Be a member of the audience for *Top Gear*
Take part in the Waendel Walk
Race a Volvo S60 around the Rockingham Race Circuit
Pay a visit to London's famous Ace Café
Sell the Mustang
Encourage someone else with a disability to do one of my
    extreme 50 List
Swim in the sea after a gap of 30 years
Go scuba diving
Travel near 160 mph in a quarter mile
Make a clay pot
Visit the capital city of Scotland

Ride a Jet Ski

Visit the capital city of Wales

Play table tennis again

Go up in a hot-air balloon

Go to the Proms

Fly an aerofoil kite

Sail a boat

Bake bread on a regular basis

Lose weight

Play more board games

Cover FIA drag-racing events in Europe for our online
   magazine

Donate funds raised through The 50 List to the CMT
   organization

Make my business work

Learn to make proper soup

~~Donate blood~~ Learn to wood turn

Go zorbing

Go to the West End of London to see a show

Pilot a narrow boat

Visit Blackpool Tower

~~Go bungee jumping~~ Learn to ski

Give a talk as a guest speaker

~~Swim 100 lengths of the local pool~~ Hand-cycle 5 miles
   uphill

Visit the capital city of Northern Ireland

Teach someone how to create a website

Complete a ~~5,000~~ 1,000-piece jigsaw puzzle

Curate a photo exhibition

THE 50 LIST

Write a comedy sketch
Write and publish a book

Not yet completed:
Spend a weekend with a Formula 1 team
Meet John Cleese
Catch a big sea fish
Get one of my photographs printed in a national
    newspaper

The reserve list (aka suggested by Ellie):
Dye my hair pink

MY COMEDY SKETCH

A Uniform Doth Not a Volunteer Make

[Fade in: ARRIVAL]

Car pulls up outside volunteer centre. Nigel releases the boot. Then he phones the centre and the lady volunteer working at her desk makes eye contact with him through the window of the centre.

NIGEL: Hello?

VOLUNTEER: Hello, can I help you?

NIGEL: Yes, I hope so. I'm sitting in the car just outside your window. I was wondering if you could help me. You see, I usually have someone with me to get my wheelchair out of the car but today I'm by myself. Can you help, please?

VOLUNTEER: Can you hold the line, please, just for a moment?

NIGEL: Yes, of course.

Volunteer covers the phone with her hand and talks to two of her colleagues, who get up and walk over to the desk to talk to her. She points Nigel out to them. They all stare at Nigel in his car.

VOLUNTEER: Hello?

NIGEL: Yes, hello?

VOLUNTEER: Sorry to keep you waiting but I'm afraid none of us can help you. You see, we're not allowed to handle wheelchairs. Goodbye.

Volunteer puts the phone down and her colleagues go back to their desks. Blinds go down. On the blinds are written the words: FRIENDLY ADVICE UP YOUR STREET.

NIGEL: But you're a volunteer centre … Hello? Hello?

Nigel looks round to see if there is anyone available to help him get his chair out from the back of the car. He sees two traffic wardens walking by. He opens the window and calls out. The first traffic warden is a tall man, George, very official looking. The second is a small man, Denis, smart but not as smart as his colleague George.

NIGEL: Hello, excuse me, can I ask you for some help, please?

GEORGE: Yes, sir. What can I do for you today?

DENIS: … do for you?

George gives Denis a disapproving look.

NIGEL: Well, my wheelchair is in the back of my car and I can't get it out myself. Can you help?

GEORGE: Oh, I would like to help you …

NIGEL: Thank you, that's very kind …

GEORGE: But I can't, I'm afraid.

DENIS: He can't.

NIGEL: You can't?

GEORGE: I can't.

NIGEL: Why not?

GEORGE: It's the uniform, you see.

NIGEL: No …

GEORGE: If I wasn't wearing this uniform, I would be more than happy to help you get your wheelchair from the back of your vehicle. But while I'm wearing this uniform I'm representing my employers, and we have strict rules when it comes to helping people lift items such as wheelchairs.

NIGEL: I just want you to get my wheelchair out for me. Is that too much to ask?

DENIS: Er, yes.

GEORGE: Look, while I'm here, do you mind if I check your Blue Badge? I'm sure it's all in order but we must check these things.

NIGEL: Yes, I suppose so.

Nigel hands his Blue Badge to the traffic warden. Seeing a photographer walking past the car, Nigel calls him over to ask him for help while George raises his glasses to inspect the disabled parking badge.

NIGEL: 'Scuse me, would you mind getting out the wheelchair from the back of my car, please?

PHOTOGRAPHER: Er, yeah, OK.

The photographer goes to the back of the car and removes the wheelchair. Inspired by its sleek lines, he places the wheelchair on the ground and starts to take photos of it. Then he puts it back in the car. Meanwhile the conversation continues between the traffic warden and Nigel.

GEORGE [*closely examining the Blue Badge to ensure the face matches the photo, with Denis looking over his shoulder*]: Mmm. Do you have any other form of identification?

NIGEL: No. Why?

GEORGE: In the photo you have a beard.

NIGEL [*distracted by what's going on behind the car with the photographer*]: Yes, but it is me. You can see that, right?

GEORGE: Oh yes, sir, but we have to look out for imposters abusing the system.

DENIS: The system …

NIGEL: Yes, I agree, but you can clearly see it's me. All I want to do is get my wheelchair out of my car and go shopping!

Nigel looks back and notices that the photographer has put the wheelchair back in the car and is leaving.

NIGEL: What's he doing? Hello?

GEORGE: I remember once a man claimed to be the owner of a Blue Badge that clearly had the image of an elderly woman on it. You can't let these people get away with it, you know.

NIGEL: Yes, indeed.

GEORGE: You see, it took all my skills and cunning to catch him out.

NIGEL [*uninterested in what George has to say*]: Really?

GEORGE: Oh yes. One of the proudest days of my life.

Nigel gives him a 'sad git' look. A van pulls up by the side of Nigel's car and a drummer gets out. He's holding drumsticks and has a towel round his neck.

NIGEL: Excuse me? Hello? Can you help me, please? Can you get my wheelchair out from the back of my car, please?

DRUMMER: Yeah, no problem, mate.

NIGEL [*feeling a little more relaxed now that he knows he's going to be able to get out of his car soon*]: Thank you.

DRUMMER: No worries.

The drummer goes to the back of the car and grabs the wheelchair. He puts it on the ground and then has the idea of using it as a wheelbarrow when he gets his drum kit out of the van.

GEORGE: Oh yes, I have seen some pretty dodgy parking in my time – like the day that ice-cream van arrived, bells clanging, and screeched to a halt on double yellows, clearly violating all parking restrictions. I was on him like a ton of bricks.

DENIS: Wasn't that an ambulance?

GEORGE: Speak when you are spoken to, Denis. Denis is in training. Anyway, you can't be too careful – these things have to be checked.

NIGEL [*trying to keep an eye on the drummer*]: How are you doing back there?

DRUMMER: OK, ta, just finishing.

The drummer has used the wheelchair to carry his equipment into a building close by and returned the wheelchair to the car.

NIGEL: What? I only wanted you to get the wheelchair out and bring it to me. Hello? Hello? (*Under his breath, as he sees that the drummer has walked off*) Where's he gone? Why's the wheelchair back in the car?

GEORGE: You see, being a traffic warden is all about keeping your eyes open. Being on the ball. I had one old lady the other day park her car without showing her Blue Badge and, harsh though it may seem, I had to give her a parking ticket.

DENIS: That was your mum, wasn't it?

GEORGE: Yes, but I had a duty to perform.

DENIS: Yes, but you had her clamped as well.

GEORGE: Serious offence calls for serious action, Denis.

DENIS: Yes, but you clamped her wheelchair!

GEORGE [*dryly*]: Thank you, Denis!

The door to the building next to the volunteer centre opens. A plumber walks out, turns and speaks to the occupants inside.

PLUMBER: I won't be long. I've just got to go and get a bit of piping to fit the radiator.

NIGEL [*seeing the plumber*]: Excuse me? Hello? Can you help me, please?

PLUMBER: Yes, mate. What can I do for you?

NIGEL: Can you get my wheelchair out from the back of my car, please?

PLUMBER: Yeah, course I can, mate. No worries.

NIGEL: Thanks.

The plumber goes to the back of the car and immediately identifies a section of the wheelchair frame that will be ideal as the piping he's looking for. He gets the chair out and starts to cut a bit out of the frame. The sound of sawing and cutting can be heard.

GEORGE: Of course, it takes several years to become a successful traffic warden. I myself have been in the job for 20 years.

NIGEL [*not interested*]: Really?

GEORGE: Oh yes, I've never missed a day.

DENIS: Weren't you suspended once?

GEORGE [*laughing nervously*]: Ha ha, Denis. Very funny.

DENIS: Yeah, you were suspended for putting a ticket on the chief constable's car.

GEORGE: He was parked illegally.

DENIS: He was on special police business, which was accompanying the mayor's limo.

NIGEL [*thinking the plumber should have got the chair out by now*]: Are you OK back there?

Silence from the back. Nigel looks around and notices that the chair is back in the car. The plumber is walking back into the building next door to the volunteer centre. As he opens the door, he speaks to the occupants.

PLUMBER: Sorted! Do you like chrome?

The plumber disappears into the building. The door closes.

NIGEL: What's going on here?

GEORGE: I'm just doing my job, sir.

NIGEL [*unaware of the damage to the wheelchair*]: No, I mean with my wheelchair. I need to get out of my car.

Just then Nigel sees a clown. He does a double take but shrugs his shoulders, as the day couldn't get any more surreal.

NIGEL: Excuse me!

The clown stops dead in his tracks and looks around to see who the voice is coming from.

NIGEL [*waving*]: Hello, over here. Me!

The clown doesn't say a word but communicates through facial expressions, hand movements and props. He looks round and sees Nigel.

NIGEL: Can you help me, please?

The clown gives a big grin and nods his head enthusiastically.

NIGEL: Great! Can you get my wheelchair out from the back of my car, please?

The clown nods again. He pulls a bunch of flowers out of his sleeve and gives it to Nigel. Then he goes to the back of the car and banging, sawing and other strange noises can be heard. Meanwhile Nigel is still putting up with jobsworth George and his boring traffic warden stories.

GEORGE: Then there was the time when I had to give a ticket to that big HGV from the Continent. If they come over here, they must know the rules of the road, y'know. It took me ages to climb up the front of the vehicle to get that ticket attached to the windscreen. But I made it.

DENIS: Yes, but the lorry driver didn't see you and pulled away with you still attached to the front of the vehicle.

GEORGE: Thank you, Denis.

DENIS: And where did you end up?

GEORGE: That's not important right now, Denis.

DENIS: Newcastle, wasn't it?

GEORGE: It was just a misunderstanding.

DENIS: Why? Did the lorry not speak English?

Nigel can't believe what he's seeing in the rear-view mirror: the clown is riding off on a unicycle. Nigel is unaware that the unicycle is made from his wheelchair.

NIGEL: What the –? I just want my wheelchair out of the car. Is that too much to ask?

Nigel sees a truck pull up next to where he is parked. The truck has the words 'SMITHS SCRAP MERCHANTS' written on the side. As the scrap man jumps down from the cab of his truck, Nigel calls him over.

NIGEL: 'Scuse me, mate. Can you help me, please?

SCRAP MAN: Yeah. Wotcha want?

NIGEL: Can you get my wheelchair out from the back of my car, please?

SCRAP MAN: I suppose so.

The scrap man goes to the back of the car. Nigel is looking hopeful that he might get his chair out of the car this time.

NIGEL: Thanks.

GEORGE: Well, must crack on. Vehicles to check, tickets to write.

DENIS [*quietly, not wanting George to hear*]: Lorries to cling to.

Once the traffic wardens have gone Nigel can open his car door. He swings his legs around in anticipation of finally getting out of the car and notices that his wheelchair is in bits and is being thrown into the scrap truck.

NIGEL: What the –?!

A single wheel that has fallen out of the boot of Nigel's car is all that is left. It rolls off down the road without him. The ladies of the volunteer centre have opened the blinds and are staring out of the windows. Nigel fixes their gaze. They close the blinds so quickly that the blinds don't come down evenly and the words on them that should read 'FRIENDLY ADVICE UP YOUR STREET' read 'UP YOUR S'.

[Fade out: THE END]

ACKNOWLEDGEMENTS

Taking on as many challenges as I did required a lot of help and I would like to acknowledge the constant support I received from a few people without whose help the task would have been that much harder.

Simon Cox was the man who said to me, after I showed him The 50 List website, 'You really must get this into the open.' Sure enough, after he made one phone call it all came to life. I'd also like to thank Simon for accompanying me on a number of the challenges, as well as making a couple of them happen.

Ian Blackett has been following me around taking photos, videos and taxiing me from one challenge to the next. His enthusiasm for what I was doing was no less than 100 per cent.

Clive Wagner edited the raw video we recorded into some really exciting pieces of work for The 50 List website, and helped me throughout.

I would also like to thank the following for their part in making some of the challenges on my list happen:

THE 50 LIST

Matt Ralph, Lucy Siegle and the rest of *The One Show*
    film crew who gave us such a memorable experience
Roy Child at Northamptonshire Sailability
James Murphy at JBSki
Shirley McLeod-Ross and her son James McLeod-Ross
    from Lagoona Park
Andy Godwin at Airkix, Milton Keynes
Mark Harris and Mike Jackson
Jeremy Palmer at Porsche Experience Centre
Caroline Day, Steve Warner, Baron Sharpe and John
    Hackney at Santa Pod Raceway
Dave Groombridge at Exclusive Ballooning
John Naude
Etam Dedhar from Bespoke Cakes By Etam
MX-5 Owners Club, Northamptonshire
My brother Gary, who taught me how to appreciate a
    single malt whisky
My brother Mark for his support and advice
My kids for letting me win occasionally
Linda Freeman
Steve Collett and Tobi Manikin-Collett at SK Motorsports
Catherine Donohoe
Rob Bibby Ceramics
Mike Donovan
Brenda Hale at Hillingdon Narrowboats Association
Sam Colby at Disability Snowsport UK
The young people at 3:16, a church youth group
My family for putting up with the puzzle on the coffee
    table all year!

Simon Cox, Julie Gray and Thomas Fegan and BNI
    Northern Ireland
Clive Wagner and Alison Pettitt
Juliet Mushen, Victoria McGeown and Lynne Barrett-Lee
Lincoln Noel Trio, the jazz band that made my 50th
    birthday party unforgettable
Mike Stokes, photographer

And finally a special mention for the CMT organization, to whom I owe so much.

CMT UK is an organization that raises awareness of the condition and works to support those who are affected by Charcot-Marie-Tooth Disease, also known as Hereditary Motor and Sensory Neuropathy or Peroneal Muscular Atrophy.

For more information, visit: http://cmt.org.uk or call 0800 652 6316 or 01202 432048

If you wish to donate money, please visit: http://www.justgiving.com/the50list